Surviving Caregiving

"Challenges of a Caregiver"

By Lois Moody RN, MS

An Xplica! Publication

ISBN 978-1501029875
ISBN 1501029878

Dedicated to John and Nicholle Moody, the Loves of My Life

&

*Healthcare Providers and Caregivers
All Very Special People*

My gratitude to my editor, Mike McHugh, without him this missive would still be sitting on the shelf. He is extraordinarily patient, kind, and intuitive.

Michael Armocida of Xplica! Publishing was extremely helpful in the final editing of this book. He is not only intuitive, but also artistic and creative. He exemplifies efficiency.

Contents

Chapter 1

Living and Dying — A Family Affair

As I looked into my daughter Nic's clear blue eyes, the same eyes I had seen since her birth 40 years previous, I experienced an emotion that I had never felt from her: deep concern.

She said that I looked frail, which was a considerable shock to me as I had never been frail or looked frail throughout my life. As a professional caregiver, my natural inclination was to be the steady source of healing and help; both in the hospital and in the home.

Nic invited me to lunch that day so we could discuss the health of the mutual love of our lives. John Moody, her father and my husband for 42 years, had been diagnosed with *idiopathic pulmonary fibrosis*. The terminal nature of his ailment had not yet sunk in for Nic; and even John refused to acknowledge the dire outlook of his condition. However as a professional caregiver, I knew that the diagnosis was bleak. I also knew that the challenges ahead would not be easy.

Living and dying is a family affair
Everyone and everything is connected. John and I were blessed with 42 years of marital bliss. We had everything that we valued: love, a beautiful daughter, harmonious home, financial security, caring

loving extended family and friends. During our life together we learned that it was better to face the problems and challenges that came our way. When John was diagnosed with pulmonary fibrosis, we decided to face that problem head-on also. We decided it would be just another season for us to endure.

Throughout life, it's natural to become accustomed to a certain way of living. Being married certainly qualifies. We couldn't imagine it any other way. Then something comes along to upset the balance and you realize that there are lots of possibilities that you just didn't see before. The question of how to handle those possibilities, and the outcomes, becomes life's greatest challenge.

Chapter 2

Symptoms and Guilt

John had always been a people person. Extremely social, everyone in our complex knew him as the fun loving and joyful person. He had been in a 'funk' for months, so I thought if we had a July 4th party he might snap out of it. John asked me not to have it, but the stubborn controlling person that I am said, "No, it will be just the thing to pick up your spirits."

John endured the party and went to bed early, which was nothing unusual over the last six months. The next morning I finally could not deny it any longer – John was sick. He went to the bathroom and came out breathing hard. He had difficultly walking to his chair. We scheduled an urgent appointment with John's primary physician.

She knew John well. With one look at him she said, "Wow, you are not the perky person that you were when I last saw you a few months ago."

Our daughter had been telling him for weeks, "We need your feisty self back... Who is this stranger?"

The lengthy diagnostic process began. Anyone who has gone through this process knows what I mean.

And now it was time to beat myself up.

How did I miss the symptoms? I am a nurse and wife. I should have known John was sick.

Guilt can play a huge role in our lives. This made John furious. He said I had been the best possible wife and mother. Give it up; the Pity Party is over.

Chapter 3

The Pity Party is Over
The Mission of this Book

I decided that the most positive thing I could do was to write about my feelings in hopes of both self-healing and healing others with similar situations. This book outlines the stages that I went through upon preempting my 'pity party,' including the progression of John's disease and how our family coped with the stages.

Sick people deserve dignity, self-esteem, and respect. Their wishes and choices should be carried out for all stages of illnesses. That was our main goal as we navigated this next season in our lives.

Additionally, I needed to let go of the anger about John's medical condition. My sanity was vital and important to my longevity. I needed to consciously remind myself that *worrying* does not take away troubles – it only takes away today's peace.

Forty plus years of nursing experience is also going to be evident in this journal. Please forgive me in advance for any biases that I may write about regarding the greatness of nurses. I am proud of my profession.

I think the best part of writing this journal was that

John read it and gave his input. It would have been so different without that communication. I am thankful that we were able to share the spirit of collaborative energy.

Chapter 4

Diagnosis of the Dis-Ease

John was diagnosed with pulmonary fibrosis in July of 2010. We were blessed to have excellent care at the VA Medical Hospital in San Diego, CA. We were also grateful that through my own professional experience and network of connections, we did not require the additional challenge of seeking authorizations for special tests, or worrying about second opinions.

After a couple months of tests, the terminal reality of John's condition started setting in. We decided to postpone further tests and lung biopsies so that we could celebrate our 42nd anniversary in Hawaii. This was the fall 2010. His condition was getting worse and more symptomatic than when he first started experiencing symptoms.

Now climbing stairs or walking any distance caused labored breathing. Travel became daunting with a new set of challenges. In our luggage we had a concentrator for Oxygen, C-pap, and a wheelchair request for the airport. Both of us felt that this was a very important family vacation. Only time would tell why.

Surviving Caregiving

Chapter 5

We are all dying

John asked our family physician if he was dying. Her response was, "We are all dying."

While this answer was shocking to both John and I, and seemed like an extremely cold, detached answer; it is clinically true. Our body parts become diseased and wear out over time. The method of adjustment to a diagnosis is our own personal decision.

In our culture, it is still viewed as taboo to discuss death. While I was a student nurse, Dr. Elisabeth Kubler-Ross gave a lecture about her groundbreaking book *On Death & Dying* at the Iowa Lutheran School of Nursing in Des Moines, IA. Her presentation and acceptance of the topic was an eye opener for me. Personally, I had not yet seen my first patient die, nor had I experienced the death of someone close to me.

In her book, Ross states, "Death is just a moment when dying ends. We have learned that for the patient, death itself is not the problem, but dying is feared because of the accompanying sense of hopelessness, helplessness, and isolation."

I knew that I would not want to be treated that way at the end of my life, nor would I want any of my loved ones dying that way.

During my second year of nurse's training an instructor gave me my only demerit. She warned that I cared too much for my patients and gave too much. She said that it would harm me later. I thought that was ridiculous.

My first patient died in 1967. She was an extremely gentle elderly woman. She asked me to read her the 23rd Psalm and then died peacefully in my arms. Thus my first experience with death was a positive one.

Chapter 6

Vacation to Ease the Stress

In September 2010, John, Nic, and I went to Oahu, Hawaii for a family vacation. It was our 42nd wedding anniversary. However the difficulties of being a tourist, stressful pace, and increased activity soon began to show in John's demeanor.

His energy levels were low, but he still wanted Nic and I to continue doing everything that we had planned. Most days he stayed at the hotel and read, or went to the pool and asked us to bring him food.

It was difficult for Nic and I to accept John's low level of participation in the vacation activities. We knew John would be very upset if we changed our plans. He emphatically told us to continue with the activities because we had come a long way and desperately needed this respite.

We were prepared for any emergency – the cell phone contained emergency numbers in case John experienced any issues. At this point, John was still doing fine.

While in Hawaii, Nic began coaching John in his pulmonary rehab. She motivated John to walk further each day. Afterwards, he would rest and read.

We started to call her the DI (Drill Instructor). When

we got back home, John began to walk and go to the pool daily, because he knew Nic was going to call. It became a joke. But whatever it took to motivate him was our ultimate goal.

~ Live life while you are healthy enough to travel. There will always be a reason to delay it: money, work, and family obligations. Be selfish and enjoy each other. Life is short.

Chapter 7

Understanding the Progression of the Disease

John next stage of diagnosis started when we got back from Hawaii. In October 2010 he had his repeat echocardiogram and spirometry.

On November 12, 2010 we had an appointment with a pulmonologist. Being a nurse makes the physician's job harder because I had acquired my own copies of the echocardiogram and spirometry and had lots of questions about both. John's lung capacity had dropped 3% and was now 49% of normal. This translates to impairment of carbon monoxide/oxygen exchange. He needed oxygen to prevent further cardiac damage. He had multiple changes in the echocardiogram.

Throughout his career in the Navy, John experienced prolonged asbestos exposure. We wondered whether the doctor would perform a biopsy, which was the only way to confirm asbestosis. The answer was, "No, it is too risky."

Because a lung biopsy could not be done, we requested that the pulmonologist consider John's asbestosis as the etiology for the fibrosis.

The pulmonologist was reluctant, and stated that he

did not know the VA system. We did not want to seek a second opinion and put John through more tests. Our daughter Nic suggested I tell the pulmonologist my concerns and maybe that would make a difference.

John's asbestos exposure was extensive from three ship overhauls without respiratory protection in the 1970-1980's. Most symptoms for asbestosis do not appear until 20-40 years post exposure.

I reviewed all of John's Navy medical records and documented his asbestosis exposure, spirometry and B reader chest X-ray results. The spirometry was normal as was the B reader chest X-ray.

John's discharge physical in 1991 stated that he had no clinical symptoms of asbestosis. However, it also noted that he had pulmonary pleural plaques and a history of asbestos exposure.

Chapter 8

Fears and Expectations

As they transition through the last stage of life, patients have many fears and expectations.

John's main fear (as his disease progressed)
Pain and suffering.

Action:
Although ultimately out of my control, I assured him that he would not suffer, whatever happened or whatever the next diagnosis would be.

John told his friend, "We thought we are invincible. We aren't."

He said that he had "turned it over to God, but God isn't ready for me yet. Que Sera, Sera – what will be, will be."

In addition to increasing feelings of helplessness, John had a total personality change since his diagnosis. I had never known John to fear anything, but after his diagnosis, he became increasingly fearful. He continually worried that he had not taken care of everything for Nic and me before his disease prevented him from doing so. This became his obsession.

He had mood swings that vacillated from angry to

very loving. John had always been a wonderful husband and father, but now he told everyone that he loved them.

When he told a friend "I love you" for the first time, we began wondering what was going on with him. He called lifelong friends and told them he loved them. He called Bob Sharp, who introduced us, and thanked him. Even his voice had changed, becoming much softer.

John's constant answer became, "I've turned it over to the Man Upstairs – God."

OK, wonderful answer, but the "Que Sera, Sera" answer was difficult for my daughter and I to accept. We wondered whether he had given up. It was confusing for us to see him so quiet and contemplative.

How much could and should we do?

John had many questions, all ending in, "Am I going to make it?" Because I am a nurse and caregiver, John grew accustomed to me having all the medical answers for 42 years, and he wanted me to reassure him that everything would be fine. But predictions are impossible and fate plays tricks on people. I did not know the answer.

The Hawaii trip was so necessary for all of us. In a few short weeks we had become exhausted: mentally, physically and spiritually. The experience left me wondering how people cope with months, even years of a family member's illness?

Chapter 9

WPMO (What Pisses Me Off!)

#1 - The diagnosis of idiopathic pulmonary fibrosis. Tabor's dictionary describes it as, "A form of interstitial lung disease, unknown etiology, with rapid deterioration in clinical course, due to diffuse fibrosis. Symptoms vary with the degree but include: dyspnea, rapid respirations, anorexia, weight loss, weakness, and fatigue – all of which were the symptoms John had experienced. As the disease progresses, finger clubbing, cyanosis, and heart failure develop

We could not say exactly when these symptoms started. I was in denial and thought John's symptoms were due to lack of exercise, deconditioning, and weight gain. But John's clothes were now loose and his symptoms persisted.

#2 - John's smoking. He smoked approximately 10 years and stopped in the 1970's, but not soon enough

#3 - Asbestos exposure while working on Navy ships. Smoking and asbestos are synergistic. Synergistic means "the action of two agents to produce a greater effect"

#4 - WPMO the most is the word " idiopathic." Idiopathic means that we did not know what was causing John's symptoms. As a respiratory therapist once said, "idio means idiot". I never liked the word before, but now I hated it

I believed his fibrosis was asbestosis, which cannot be confirmed without a lung biopsy. The risk of a lung biopsy was too great and the diagnosis would not change the course of the illness – so my anger was futile.

As an Occupational Health Nurse with the Navy for 25 years, I gave hundreds of lectures about asbestos exposure, prevention, and medical surveillance. I made shipboard visits and taught medical personnel about all aspects of prevention of asbestosis, yet I could not prevent my husband's exposure and subsequent diagnosis.

#5 - John – for not exercising. He was going to the pool and walking, and I hoped that was enough. The pulmonary rehab taught him what he needed to do to help maintain the lung function he had

#6 - Impulsive car buying. *Car Country Carlsbad* and all dealerships worldwide love John and John–wannabes. I'm sure John owned at least a hundred cars in his lifetime. If there was any mystery in John's personality, for me it was this one. I distinctly remember a few weeks after we were married, John came home and gleefully hollered, "Honey, what you are doing?" Scrubbing the bathroom floor was my answer.

How do I remember? Because I came to hate that question, it usually meant there was a different car in our driveway

The first car was a Polaris, a block long yellow and black bumblebee. I blocked most cars that John bought from my memory bank. But another car was just as memorable. He bought me a lime green Javelin. Why in God's name? I asked. I am sure that I had a perfectly serviceable car before that one. At the time, I was a Public Health Nurse in Boone, IA. Not a stealth job for sure, but it also was not good when the rumor in this small town came to my attention. One of my patients had a positive TB test and I had to follow up his meds and treatment.

Sometimes it is just not smart to meet some patients where they live, thus his suggested meeting place was the pub below his apartment. Not ideal, but better than being alone with him. Or so I thought, until I walked into my office and Irene, the other nurse laughingly asked if I knew what the newest rumor was in Boone. I responded, no. We lived in Des Moines 40 miles away, so why would I care about rumors in Boone? The rumor was; this alcoholic patient was having an affair with the nurse who drove the lime green car. I was the only nurse with such a car. I came to hate that car. Everyone in Boone knew who I was, where I was, whom I was visiting and how long I was there. Lime green cars in small Iowa towns are not the best image for a Public Health Nurse.

When John read this paragraph, he smiled and said, "Well it hasn't been boring." No indeed.

When family or friends wanted to start a little trouble between us, they would say, "Gee, John haven't you had this car a long time?"

Car negotiating and buying energized John, which was one of the great mysteries of my life.

However in October 2010 he had my blessing. He had the Cadillac three years, an eternity for John. Nic was coming to have breakfast with John and then they were going car shopping. She did contract negotiation in her job, so she already knew how to negotiate but her father would add to that knowledge.

John knew that Nic the DI was coming that day, so he put his oxygen on and walked several blocks, followed by pool-walking and the Jacuzzi.

These days I was encouraging John to do anything that energized him. Another thing that I've never understood is casinos and gambling. But I remember encouraging John to call his friend Ted and go to the casino. Nic was very surprised when she heard this. I saw John sitting around watching TV non-stop and being depressed. He was shocked when I suggested it and asked why.

I wanted him to get out of the house and do something he enjoyed. John would not jeopardize our financial security, and a few hours with his friend would be good therapy.

Did I still want John to be the impulsive car buyer that made me so angry over the years? I did not know, but John was becoming someone I did not recognize. He was exhausted and started regularly turning down dinner invites from friends.

John retired to bed early these days, sometimes 6pm. He read before falling asleep. John was not using his oxygen through this car buying process, so I was concerned that his body was probably physiologically decomposing.

After reading this, you may surmise that I am a really "pissed off" person. Not so, but I guess there was a lot of negativity sitting in the cobwebs of my brain.

No more. If we live a rich full life, unhappiness sadness and anxiety are going to be part of it. We all have a bewildering potpourri of emotions: Love, anger, tenderness, bitterness, rage, and quiet calm. I do not have the energy or desire to focus on negative – self-defeating things, thus they all have to go. My mental, physical, and spiritual health is too vital to me.

Self-reflection is always good. When you journal, or write about a topic, it can help prevent you from going "round and round" in circles rehashing worries, which is counter-productive.

I was angry, but had to give myself permission to be angry so that I could let it go. I was angry with God, but thought she could deal with it.

I was angry at John's illness and the possibility of losing my life's partner.

~ Denial/reality is interchangeable sometimes. We see and hear what we want to.

Reality is more evident when you are the daily caregiver. Nurses know too much and not enough. But I read the echocardiogram and spirometry reports and it was hard not to speculate about the future.

Add D to anger and it becomes DANGER. Beware signal for us.

Chapter 10

Pulmonary Rehabilitation

John started his Pulmonary Rehab at UCSD on Oct 18, 2010. He walked in without using his oxygen and swiftly received a lecture on the importance of oxygen.

The staff at the UCSD Pulmonary Rehab department was so dedicated and inspiring. The staff helped John understand how the fibrosis was causing his symptoms, and they also helped him set goals. He was told (gently) that it would not be possible to regain a portion of his lung capacity. They agreed that his goals should be to maintain current lung function and increase his strength and endurance with continuous purposeful exercise.

Pulmonary fibrosis is a disease that plays havoc with the psyche. The patient becomes frustrated when he has to stop any activity because he can't breathe. The rehab helped John see that he was not alone, and hopefully helped him accept his limitations with less frustration.

Knowledge is definitely powerful. Rehab taught him the three P's of breathing: posture, pacing yourself, and breathing with pursed lips. Also that it is important to engage the diaphragm to assist with lung inflation of oxygen. When the lungs are fibrotic, they are scarred and stiff. They cannot move as much to oxygen. Pursed lip breathing is important for slow and easy, unforced breathing. Planning ahead and pacing oneself allows for the conservation of energy. Bending over compresses the lungs, thus simple activities like tying ones shoes will cause shortness of breath.

After the training sessions, the physical portion of the rehab began. Vitals were taken prior to the exercise. In John's case, his pulse was only 40, which concerned the therapist.

My response surprised her, "I know he has bradycardia (slow pulse), and has had it for years." She hesitated then asked if it was really safe for him to continue. I reassured her that it was. She asked me not to leave and returned to the exercise room. Thirty minutes later and while he was on the treadmill, his pulse finally climbed to 60.

On December 1, 2010, the Pulmonary Rehab addressed 'Panic Control', causes of respiratory distress, symptoms and physical body reactions. Steps to manage symptoms were discussed, including pacing oneself to prevent respiratory distress. This is easier said than done.

Activity should be stopped immediately when symptoms arise. Pursed lip breathing, body positions, and relaxation techniques should all be tried prior to oxygen for breathlessness or labored breathing.

Tips for proper use of oxygen equipment:

- When using oxygen, stay 5 ft away from matches, candles, cigarettes, gas burners, fireplaces

- Keep oxygen units 5 ft from space heaters, steam pipes, furnaces, radiators

- Keep oxygen out of direct sunlight

- Turn off oxygen completely when not in use

Do Not Do list:

- Do not smoke and don't allow others to smoke in the home

- Do not use vapor rubs, petroleum, and oil based hand lotions as they are flammable. Use water based products only

- Do not oil the oxygen unit or use with greasy hands

- Do not use aerosol sprays, air fresheners, and hair sprays, which are very flammable

- Do not use oxygen while cooking with gas

- Do not place the liquid oxygen canisters on their side. The liquid inside may evaporate

The class 'Traveling with Chronic Lung Disease' was another eye-opener. During this session, I realized that John had pulmonary problems for at least 12 years. The disease involves a gradual onset with increasing difficulty breathing.

Hindsight is always 20/20. We had taken several trips to high altitudes. The first trip John had respiratory problems was in Vail, Colorado in 1998. We stopped there on a cross-country trip. As we were walking, John said, "I am going back to the hotel, I don't feel well." I walked with him back to the hotel. He complained of shortness of breath. He did not have chest pain or cardiac symptoms, which was my first concern because he had a family history of heart problems.

John wanted me to see the city, so I went for a short walk and returned to the hotel. He was still short of breath. Again I attributed it to deconditioning, weight gain, lack of exercise and high altitude. We decided not to risk it and returned to lower altitude.

The 2nd trip with respiratory issues was in December 2000. John met Nic and I in Lake Tahoe for her 30th birthday. She and I were having a marvelous time. John had been in Iowa for his sister Betty's kidney transplant.

When John arrived, he was tired and grouchy, which we thought was attributed to his long trip. However, that night I awakened Nic and told her we had to leave because John was experiencing shortness of breath. He had no other symptoms. His pulse and blood pressure were normal.

The third trip was in 2002 while we were in the foothills of Yellowstone Park in Wyoming. John was experiencing shortness of breath, so we left and returned to Carlsbad, California. Note: This is SEA LEVEL. During this period of time John had numerous cardiac evaluations, but no chest x-rays. The medical profession decided that chest x-rays cause too much radiation exposure. As a nurse I feel this decision has prevented a lot of early disease identification. In John's case, however, I do not believe that it would have impacted the outcome.

Surviving Caregiving

Chapter 11

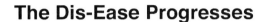

The Dis-Ease Progresses

John graduated from Pulmonary Rehab on December 8, 2010. The discharge summary indicated John's progress: He increased his treadmill walking speed and time, his perceived "breathlessness" stayed at the level 2.

Recommendations were:

- Continue walking at a pace of up to 2.5 mph/grade as tolerated

- Use continuous oxygen with heavy exercise

- Mid-setting on oxygen conserving device with light exercise

John renewed his gym membership instead of returning to the maintenance program at UCSD, which was 35 miles away.

By Christmas 2010 John was using more oxygen and his breathing was more labored.

When you live with someone, daily changes are not obvious; but our family members noticed that John was having more difficulty breathing. Additionally, John asked me if I thought that it would be his last Christmas.

How do you respond to that question? I didn't have a clue, but I blew it off and vowed to make it the best Christmas ever.

The symptoms appeared to be more loss of lung capacity. We had several days of heavy rains. As they said in Pulmonary Rehab, when the weather is "soupy" it is harder to breathe.

When it was not raining, John would exercise at the gym or the pool. He was always extremely fatigued and needed more oxygen after these sessions, but he knew that he had to do it to maintain his lung capacity, strength, and endurance. He was doing his best, but it was hard to watch.

Christmas came filled with love, joy, giving, sharing, and eating. Our family togetherness was so special, and numerous friends brought us cookies and other goodies. Everyone was saddened when they saw the physical changes in John.

He expended most of his energy trying to be the fun loving, mischievous person everyone remembered; but he had to stop and use oxygen. After visitors left, he collapsed in bed with the concentrator (oxygen) and C-pap.

Dealing with a progressive disease was emotionally taxing for both the patient and the family. BUT WE WERE SO BLESSED WITH FAMILY AND FRIENDS and knew that we were not alone on this journey.

Chapter 12

Being Grateful

Gratefulness – a unique look at our lives.

What my husband and I shared:

#1 - Mutual love and respect

#2 - Our daughter Nic – the love of our lives

#3 - Support of each other's dreams

#4 - A life in San Diego

#5 - Our happy, healthy, harmonious home

#6 - Financial planning for comfort, safety, and security

#7 - My nursing degree, which is precious to me

When I was twenty-four, I was accepted at Iowa Lutheran School of Nursing in Des Moines. I graduated and passed the boards in 1967 and began my 40-year plus nursing career. Eventually, I earned my BS and MS. This was truly a family affair. My husband typed term papers and my daughter did chores to keep the home front smooth so I could work full time, go to school, and have family time. I worked as an

Occupational Health Nurse for the Navy and traveled from Spain to Whidbey Island. I also visited all military hospitals in the US to evaluate Occupational Health programs. I worked seven years after my retirement from civil service for the Department of Labor in Workers Compensation Nurse Case Management.

#8 - Friends, also precious, frequently help us in rough times. A dear friend sent me an email, which greatly helped. In part it said:

When God takes something from your grasp he's not punishing you but merely opening your hands to something better. The will of God will never take you where the Grace of God will not protect you.

It goes on to say:

There comes a point in your life when you realize: Who matters? Who never did? Who won't anymore?

And who always will. So, don't worry about people from your past, There's a reason why they didn't make it to your future.

I recently read an interview article with Michael J Fox. He said he does two things every day – he is always accepting and grateful. Incredible!!!!!

Each day that John and I had together was special. I was so happy that I had retired so we were able to share quality time together.

Chapter 13

Feeling Useless

January 6, 2011

John was having a bad day and was obsessing again that he was a useless. While I was talking on the phone with a friend, John stormed out and slammed the door. I ended the conversation, cried, and called Nic to see if she was free for lunch. She could tell I was having a bad day.

When the patient is having a bad day, the caregiver is having a worse day. I took a long bath, then got coffee and a pedicure to relax.

Nic and I went for Mexican food and, for me, a two-margarita lunch. Nic knew exactly what was happening. Her social work background was a lifesaver during these days. She listened to me vent. She told me that if I could not set limits for myself, I would get sick. This I already knew, but she was ready to take drastic measures, including calling my family and friends and asking them not to share anything with me that was not positive.

It is true that I have a terrible time setting limits for myself, and many times I take on everyone else's problems. During this time, I contemplated a new title for this book - *Staying sane while caregiving.*

Caregivers must receive as well as give. This is probably hard if you are a caregiver.

Chapter 14

Caregiver Characteristics

I would like to preface this section by repeating what someone told me recently, "If we love the person we are caring for, then we have to love them enough to take care of ourselves first, so we have the health and energy to care for our loved ones."

It is great advice, but try putting that into practice. It is much easier said than done, as you will see throughout this book.

I have probably been a caregiver since I was age 18 months. I am the oldest of 6 children, except for an older brother, who did not live with us until we were teenagers. From that early age I was responsible for helping mom care for my siblings and other associated duties.

I have always been first to assist family members when they are ill. I have done this not out of obligation but because I always wanted to help. Additionally, I have always been the first called when there was a family issue. My brother Johnny continuously warned me that I cannot take on everyone's problems. Did I ever listen? Never. I am stubborn. Stubbornness can be a great quality by the way.

I have been blessed with lots of energy and a wonderful husband and daughter who understood and always supported me when I had to do whatever I could to help others.

John would say that I should start my own soup kitchen because I made soup for neighbors and other people who were ill.

I am usually the person called if there is a medical emergency in our condo complex. Again, these are things I am qualified for and enjoy doing. But they symbolize the caregiver role.

Sometimes I think that I must have a huge C on my forehead. I recently walked to the ocean and when I returned I stopped at a garage sale. There were several books that I would have bought if I had money with me. The lady said, "Come back, I will save them for you." I declined the offer and explained that I was taking my husband to the hospital for an appointment.

She looked closer at me and said, "Oh my God, you are the caregiver." She gave me a warm hug and asked if I was doing anything for myself.

She proceeded to tell me her caregiving story. Millions of people have them. Her husband suffered a lengthy illness and had both legs amputated for peripheral circulation caused from smoking. She would wake up at 5am, drive 35 miles to work, and then come home and care for her husband. This lasted several years.

She said that when he died fourteen years prior,

people said, "How sad." But her response was, "No it wasn't. Neither of us had a life and he did not want to continue to live being a burden to me."

It is so true that if you listen to other people, then you will realize that many others have it worse. This made me appreciate my life in comparison to her caregiver challenges.

Another friend, Sheila, was caregiver for her husband Nicky when he died. She was also caring for their quadriplegic son. One day I visited her and brought them soup. She had just returned from having a manicure. At the time I thought that was very strange. But now I understood that she needed a short respite to continue her caregiving duties.

Caregivers always neglect personal health and needs to put others first. Respite is so important, as it helps to recharge the batteries to care for another.

This will be different for each individual. Whatever it is, do it without guilt. If the caregiver becomes sick, who will care for the already ill person?

However, it is hard to practice what I preach.

Surviving Caregiving

Chapter 15

Emotional Landmines

Week of January 10, 2011

We were at the VA twice this week. I was reviewing all of John's medical records to challenge the VA on John's diagnosis. I knew that they would not easily accept the claim of asbestosis with just the pulmonologist's letter. The VA is overwhelmed with claims from the military people returning from the wars. John's case was not the highest priority.

I had all of John's reports since his new diagnosis and researched adjudications for asbestosis. We submitted a 25-page document highlighted and underlined. Only time would tell if the claim would be accepted. However, it is extremely important to do the research and submit a succinct package.

The previous week, my daughter and I both noticed a significant deterioration in John's condition. His appointment with the pulmonologist on January 21, 2011, proved our anxieties were well founded. The VA is a teaching hospital, so we saw a resident who was not familiar with John. I had reviewed the report from John's lung perfusion/vent imaging and asked the resident to explain the meaning of the statement "Evidence of bilateral perfusion inhomogeneity, predominately non-segmental in appearance."

The resident, unaccustomed to family members descending upon him with medical reports and requesting answers, seemed overwhelmed. After reviewing the case history, he left to consult with his advisor.

Dr. F, who had previously been treating John, came in next. Nic told him that we were all a "train wreck". She and I both were crying and John was terrified (not stated of course). Dr. F compassionately told us John's disease had progressed rapidly, and John needed to get his affairs in order.

Dr. F said when John's breathlessness symptoms were not controlled with his current oxygen that a "trans tracheal procedure" could be performed to administer oxygen directly into the lungs. Dr. F told us he does not like the procedure and John rejected it.

John then asked him how long he had the condition, and whether it was related to asbestos exposure.

Dr. F told us he really hated this disease. John said, "Not as much as I do." At this point it did not matter what the diagnosis was, the outcome would be the same.

We then proceeded into the *emotional landmines*. Dr. F patiently listened through a heated family discussion about John's psychiatric care. John loved his psychiatrist, but Nic and I did not think he understood the level of John's depression. Dr. F observed all of this.

John adamantly stated he would not change psychiatrists – end of conversation. The patient rules.

Dr. F finally told Nic that we could seek other psych referrals if we chose and that he could facilitate Hospice Care when the time came.

The next recommendation shocked all of us. Up to this point, we thought Dr. F had no sense of humor – not so. He said there was one drug that John could try. He then said the generic name of Viagra. The doctor and John smiled at each other.

Dr. F turned to me and said, "I will give you a broom to fight him off." Nic had a very dramatic response, "Mom, give him a little and he will be cured." After the laughter we asked if he was serious, "Yes, Viagra improves the blood flow to the lungs as well as the rest of the body." No wonder the TV add is so effective. Viagra will be prescribed twice a day. WHOA.

Surviving Caregiving

Chapter 16

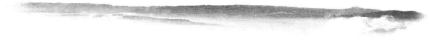

DNR

January 28, 2011

John had an appointment with his primary care physician. He called to request this appointment after he knew that I was going to be with Nic at the same time. This was so unlike John. After the appointment he told me, "It went well. She wants to meet with you and take the Trust with the DNR (Do not resuscitate) and end of life decisions. He also told me Dr. H would coordinate the Hospice and anything else that needed to be done.

The visit puzzled me. John always wanted me with him at his appointments to interpret the medical lingo. However, it was absolutely his right to see physicians privately. John had a one and a half hour session scheduled with his psychiatrist. This was usually a thirty-minute session max. I was glad John has this outlet and hoped he discussed his anger and depression. But again, that was personal and private. He asked if he should go to Dr. F's superior for medical review and second opinion.

This was John's decision and I asked if he wanted to start all over with tests, evaluations, and histories. His answer was "No." All three of us saw John's changes/deterioration. I wanted the time that John had left and his energy spent doing what he wanted to do.

A card framed in our living room says:

Live in harmony with the changing seasons

See the beauty each one offers

Hear the song each one sings to your heart

And celebrate every age for its own joys and discoveries

During the first week of February, several of John's life-long friends visited. It was joyful and sad at the same time.

Chapter 17

Hospice and Palliative Care

Hospice: Team of Compassion (for Life's Conclusion)

Hospice is the most compassionate team approach to end of life issues. The team consists of the patient, family, physicians, nurses, social workers, spiritual advisors, aides, and volunteers. The team develops a palliative plan to assist the patient in the journey to next stage.

The purpose of hospice is to relieve or alleviate symptoms without curing the patient. Comfort and pain control are the goals. We no longer worry about patients being addicted to meds when they die. Before hospice that was actually a concern.

Hospice personnel also assist the family with understanding the stages of *end of life transition.*

I had to trust my intuition. It was difficult for me as a wife/nurse not to speculate about John's possible outcomes. Sometimes nurses know too much, yet not enough to have all the answers.

We had an appointment with the social worker to discuss end of life issues for John. He updated his medical power of attorney and Advanced Directive stating he wanted "maximum comfort but no life saving measures."

This was a necessary but stressful experience. The social worker also wrote a letter to the VA Regional office stating John was given 6-12 months to live and requested the VA to expedite the claim for fibrosis/asbestosis. She also attached the medical report from Dr. F (dated 1/21/11), which showed John's rapid declining medical status.

We discussed palliative and hospice care. The emphasis of The San Diego VA Palliative Care Unit was: the best quality of life for the patient and family for chronic non-curable diseases and to provide diligent pain and symptom management.

Generally, the interdisciplinary hospice team includes: doctors, nurses, chaplains, and dieticians. This unit also has End of Life Care Beds for veterans with anticipated 2-3 week life expectancy. These beds are limited and dependent on the VA disability rating. Only those with 70% service connected disability are eligible for this unit. John had 90% disability. He requested a notation be made in his record that he chose this facility for his last weeks of life.

Nic and I protested that he should be at home, but he was insistent that we needed the help and support. Admission to this unit is determined on a case-by-case basis and availability of beds.

February 4

We received a call from the palliative care nurse and he reviewed John's symptoms and made an appointment for us to see the team physician on February 11. During this phone consult he asked about John's breathlessness. It had increased and was becoming especially obvious when he got up to use the bathroom.

The nurse asked if anyone had recommended 'low dose opiates'. They had found that low doses of morphine tricks the brain into thinking it needs less oxygen. That made so much sense to me. Additionally, it met our goal for John to improve his comfort and quality of life.

I was trying to let go of my control issues and accept John's request for admission to the palliative care unit when we needed it. I always expected he would be at home for his last days. John again showed his compassion for Nic and I and wanted us to accept all available help. Nic had been advised that she needed to stay positive for John and not cry or show her emotions about John's decline.

John's response was, "I would be a little upset if you were not upset about me right now." So true!

We had always been a sharing, caring family. So denial and trying to hide our emotions would not work for long. Sooner or later, one of us would pick up on it and challenge the other to be honest and express true feelings. Thank God for this or it all would have been even more difficult.

Thankfully Nic and I had alternated days of 'losing it', which included crying, anger, frustration, being short fused and saying things we would never dream of saying at another time, withdrawing, trying to protect each other when we were really depressed, fatigued, and mentally and physically exhausted. We knew that these emotions were normal for this period in our lives but that did not take away the feeling.

Nic stayed with us several days, which gave all of us the opportunity to rebalance as much as possible. We were so blessed to have our family togetherness. Nic and John shared a love of TV detective, law and order types of programs and she frequently called John to tell him about a new show. She would program the TV to record shows to watch during her next visit. The sharing was so wonderful to watch and hear the delight in John's voice when Nic called to discuss the shows.

We treasured the time we had left with John and tried to be at peace with our lives and our future, whatever it would hold.

I had known the signs of burnout for a long time and thought we might be at risk. We would have to watch for this. I only knew one thing for sure: Nic and I still had too much to live for. I did not know what the future held, nor did I have control over it, and would not want to.

We would need to meet each challenge and adjust to it, whatever it was. I would have to learn to ask for help and accept it. That would be another challenge for me. My independence was one of my most valued strengths. We had never been in this position before. Yes, we had lost loved ones as has everyone, but we had never lost my husband or Nic's father. It was a terrifying experience for us.

Surviving Caregiving

Chapter 18

Red Velvet Cake

John always loved the pool. It was his sanctuary. He pool-walked when he could and then would relax and meditate in the sun and Jacuzzi. This was so important for his mental and physical stamina.

Unfortunately he did not take his oxygen with him, which was a source of frustration for me. I knew and respected his pride, but he would return from the pool very breathless and then would sit to recoup with oxygen in his chair. I did not nag him about this, but it was difficult to watch. It was important for his independence to keep going for as long as he could.

February 8

John had extremely labored breathing after he walked to the bathroom and returned to bed. He said, "The pool-walking is not helping is it?"

I contemplated how to answer – either lie to him for encouragement or be truthful? Truth won out. We both cried.

The next morning, John did not have any early morning appointments, but he was still fatigued after 10 hours of sleep.

John had a fondness, more like an obsession, for Red Velvet cake and cupcakes. He got whatever he wanted these days, so 4pm every day he had the cake and ice cream. His appetite had diminished. Then he would go to bed and read.

February 11

We had an appointment at the Palliative Care facility of the VA Hospital. The mission of this department is symptom and comfort control. This met our objective for John.

Early on I promised John that I would attempt to control his pain and discomfort. If I ever needed a lesson in letting go of control, this was it.

We met with the doctor in charge of the clinic. After an extensive conversation with us, he recommended Vicodin for John's breathlessness.

Research has shown that opiates are now the Standard of Care for patients with pulmonary problems. The doctor emphasized the importance of John avoiding anyone who would be infectious as his immunity was compromised.

Repeatedly, the doctor emphasized John's quality of life, not quantity. The Vicodin would hopefully decrease John's anxiety. When we are anxious our breathing is significantly affected. John continually denied his apprehension to Nic. However John tried to be funny during our discussion with the physician; which was a true indicator of John's real apprehension.

John's energy, mentally and physically, was waning after our meeting. John and Nic had the same reaction to this appointment. Both were angry and did not want it to be reality. Nic and John both reacted to the palliative care unit's environment. Nic told me that I needed to Feng Shui it. They did not see the compassion or empathy of the healthcare providers.

Again, I told John that when his end of life came that we should keep him at home with hospice assistance. John did not understand any of this and he kept saying that he did not want to be a burden and for our last memories to be of him dying.

Another concern arose – John was a gun collector. I was worried about John's depression and his continuous statement that he would not be a burden to me at his end of life. John had previously been suicidal. Maybe I over reacted, but I wanted to have the guns out of the house. My daughter and I were undecided ... should we remove the shells? Should we have a friend remove them?

Incredibly, as I was agonizing about the guns, John asked what I would think if he gave the guns away this week to friends and family who were visiting. I was so grateful I began to cry with relief. Everyone was pleased with his or her gifts. Apparently one was an expensive antique.

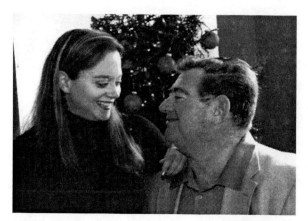

Dedication

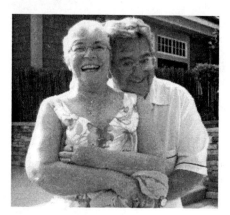

Marital bliss

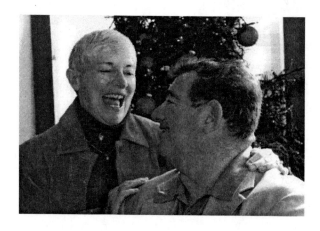

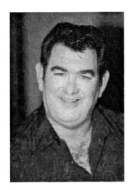

Car buying

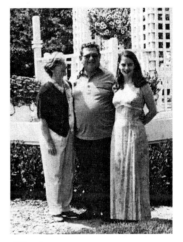

Christmas

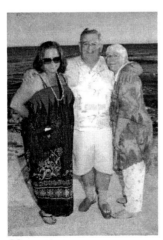

Vacation

Surviving Caregiving

Chapter 19

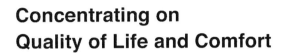

Concentrating on
Quality of Life and Comfort

February 11

It was beautiful here. My friend and I met for a walk and John joined us for her birthday lunch. I needed the exercise, ocean, relaxation and time to breathe myself before we got a house full of very well meaning family members. Their love and compassion were so valued. They were all taking our energy into consideration and only staying a few days each.

Until this time, I never understood how people could become addicted to Vicodin or other opiates. Now I did. John had three days of ½ pill twice a day and his breathing was deeper, less labored, and his stamina for visitors was high.

We really enjoyed having everyone visit. He slept 8-10 hours at night and took a nap during the day. He was less anxious and had more energy. Who cares if he was addicted at this stage of his life? Quality and comfort were our goals.

Week of February 13

Our home was filled with relatives. It was a joyous week of love, laughter, tears and reminiscing. We got to spend time with nieces and nephews. Nic was working from home that week, so she was able to get reacquainted with her cousins.

We felt tremendously blessed with our wonderful caring, loving family. That is what families are for – to love and support each other through the good and the bad times.

Chapter 20

Letting go of Possessions

February 21

All the visitors had departed. I was asleep when John woke me and asked me to take his pulse. It was rapid for him and irregular. He was having labored breathing and was very anxious. He had taken ½ Vicodin 30 minutes before this episode. I gave him another ½ Vicodin, increased his oxygen level, and massaged his back with lavender baby oil. He was able to relax and go to sleep. It was very frightening for both of us.

During this time we were both exhausted. John was sleeping eight to ten hours at night with long naps during the day. This bothered him significantly. He could not understand why he had no energy and was exhausted with very little walking, even with the oxygen.

He said, "I am getting weaker, aren't I?" We discussed the fibrosis, his lack of oxygen, and the medications. They all contributed to his fatigue/exhaustion.

John asked me again what I would do with the life insurance money. That answer was always the same – pay off the condo of course. It was getting easier to answer that question. I did not know if he forgot that we had discussed this issue at least a thousand times or what other possible explanation there was for this question.

He was obsessing. Repeatedly stating that he had not done enough for Nic and me financially. I knew we would be fine. Fortunately we had planned for this stage of life. My constant reassurances did not appease him. These conservations always left me exasperated.

John had always been a good provider for both Nic and I. For some reason he could not accept that. We had worked together as a team to create a wonderful family, home, paradise. What more could we want? John's health yes, but we had no control over what was happening. It was honest and hard to accept.

February 23

John sold his Rolex watch and gave away a leather coat that I bought for him 40+ years ago. Again, I had to ask, "Is he letting go and is that the same as giving up?"

February 26

John's sleep was becoming restless and he was having a recurring dream/nightmare of drowning. We decided to increase his Vicodin to a whole pill at night. It was 3am and I, the insomniac, was awake while John was sleeping like a baby. The whole pill of Vicodin worked.

Chapter 21

Finding Peace in the Final Days

The week of February 27th included many soul searching and intense discussions between John and I. John was anxious and deeply concerned that when he died it would be painful. I assured him that the meds would prevent any pain. He was pain free at that point.

Also, John did not look ill. In fact he had lost weight and people would comment that he couldn't be that sick. Additionally, John was always expending his energy when people were around and then collapsing after they left.

On February 28 two friends (Sheila and Helen) brought John a prayer blanket. Sheila's husband Nicky died 2 years ago. Sheila had kept him at home with the help of hospice. This week I told John that I wanted him to die at home. He thought it would be too hard on me. I called the Palliative Care Unit at VA and we planned to meet with them after an appointment with the pulmonologist on March 4.

Sheila was a great help in reassuring John that I could handle his dying at home with hospice assistance.

When John and I were discussing his fears he asked me if he would drown, as in his nightmares. I told him that I could not lie to him, but assured him that there were meds to relieve these symptoms. I believe people wait for loved ones to release them to "go in peace." It would be harder with John. But we promised him that he would "die with dignity."

March 2

John's oxygen was delivered. I asked the driver if his company provided DME (durable medical equipment) such as hospital beds, etc. when it became necessary. Our complex was difficult to get into, so I thought pre-planning would be wise. John's TV/ reading room would be easily adaptable when we needed the equipment. It was distressing to John that I had thought this out and had a plan. I also thought that it probably reassured him. But the reality was that the disease was progressing rapidly.

Chapter 22

Hospice Begins

Oh My God - what an incredibly long day March 4 was! We started with the pulmonologist.

In general, doctors always want to find a cure, and sometimes they do not accept that patients will die. I think this appointment was as difficult for Dr. F as it was for John and I.

He performed the history and chest exam. John still had 'rales' at the base of his lungs. No surprise there. The doctor increased John's Viagra to 3 times/day. Drugs would not save John and everyone in the room knew it, but if seeing a patient deteriorate is difficult for a doctor, then what the hell do you think it is like for the patient and family?

John said he wanted 2 more years to live. Dr. F said we were doing the right thing with hospice at home and he thought John had a few more months. Doctors are not God and cannot predict the future with certainty, but John was deteriorating. The next stop was palliative care.

Thank you God for nurses.

When I told Michael, the nurse in charge, about John's nightmare of drowning and suffocating, he pulled up a chair in the hallway and told John that he could not count the number of times patients had this dream. He said, "No, dying is not like that. There are meds to alleviate those anxieties."

I was so relieved. A fellow nurse knew exactly what to say. Michael gave me a long hug.

John was becoming increasingly frustrated and went to see the Veteran's Rep to see if he could expedite the VA claim for asbestosis. The answer was no. The case was still before the board. But John being the head of the family needed to make sure that Nic and I were taken care of. Michael agreed that the *end of life* should be at home if possible.

We discussed the available hospice agencies in our area and agreed on Elizabeth Hospice. Michael made a phone call at 3pm for an intake appointment for 4pm. God, what a relief. The intake hospice nurse arrived. John missed his nap that day but we felt so relieved to know that John, Nic, and I would not be making the *end of life* journey alone.

I knew we had resources available and was aware of the benefits of hospice. But until we experienced it, we did not fully comprehend the relief.

There is nothing like hospice visits to make you reassess your life. Again, I asked John if there was anything that he wanted to do. The answer was consistent, "No, we have done everything and have everything."

The hospice nurses were wonderful. We reviewed John's medications and symptoms. I was told that I could give John the drug Ativan if he had another panic attack. Additional meds were discussed for later usage. John's history was reviewed, and he really connected with the nurses.

Rarely did John offer his addiction, Red Velvet cake, to anyone, but he did on March 7. John and the nurses ate and laughed. John's wicked sense of humor charmed everyone. I told the nurses that he would be funny until his last breath – I prayed that would be true. I would hate to see that change. Both nurses left saying that it would be great to work with us.

Later, Ted, John's friend, called to arrange their Tuesday morning breakfast. They agreed to go to the casino afterwards. John told me, "I don't know how many more times I will be able to do that."

The reality was that we did not know how long his energy would allow him to go out. He needed to enjoy every minute. Tuesday morning he left with a full tank of oxygen. I gave him an extra Vicodin if his breathlessness became severe and told him to definitely take one on the trip home.

Surviving Caregiving

Chapter 23

Period of Lasts

I think that March 9 was the beginning of our period of *lasts*. A friend of mine told me when her husband died she was told there would be a year of *firsts* – such as first birthday, first holiday without her husband, etc. This was our period of *lasts.*

John came home from the casino absolutely exhausted, watched a little Fox news and went to bed. He was extremely anxious with labored breathing. I gave him a quarter tablet of Ativan. He had already taken a Vicodin. I gave him a lavender oil massage and his oxygen. He went to sleep.

No sleep for me. I had projects waiting to be done, as always. John was asleep so I got up and started new project. After finishing, sleep still evaded me. I had taken an herbal sleep aid that I got from an acupuncturist. After eight months of being the daily caregiver, I knew that I must again change my ways or there would be two sick patients. I could not allow that to happen.

Damn, this was hard. I was going to have to get some quality sleep. Additionally, I was past due for my annual mammogram. When I called to schedule the mamo the receptionist said, "It has been two years since you have seen Dr. R. You will have to have a physical first." OK, I had neglected my health, so made an appointment for next week.

When John briefly woke up after 12 hours of sleeping, he said, "My time of playing with the big boys is over isn't it?" When I asked what that meant, he said that he didn't want to believe Dr. F that he only had a few months to live, but thought he must be right. We both cried. He did not know I had been crying most of the night, because when he came back yesterday it was obvious that the fun day was also an exhausting day. Plus he was coughing and sneezing. The smoke at the casino was not helpful, but it was not my job to tell John that now. I wanted him to enjoy every minute, no matter what it was. "Quality, not quantity of life is so important now."

Yes, there is a non-smoking area at the casino but you have to walk through the smoking area. The smoke filters throughout the casino.

It is obvious I am a non-smoker and I have to tell you it was hard when smokers came to see John. Even though they would smoke outside, it still penetrated their clothes. I would always ended up with a sore throat, psychological or what I did not know, but did not need it.

Enough of my preaching; John had been asleep for 15 hours. After our talk he turned over and went back to sleep. It looked like he had a significant facial change, his eyes looked sad and his mouth drooped. He said, "I love you and Nic, and thank you for being so sweet and taking care of me." That broke my heart. Resignation had set in. I did not think of myself as sweet, but knew how much he appreciated the life we had together.

Surviving Caregiving

Chapter 24

Rhythm of Life

The next hospice appointment was with Pat, our spiritual advisor. We spent two delightful hours with her. We immediately connected with Pat. It was reminiscent of the teachings of Taoism, which explains connections between people with each other and to the environment. John connected with her from his religious values and me from my spiritual side. Tao expresses what the Chinese accept and call the *Rhythm of Life*.

Carl Jung wrote that intuition and synergy are powerful forces in our lives. As terrible as John's situation was, I firmly believed God had placed Pat and the hospice team in our lives to help us traverse this period. Pat believed in the teachings of Elizabeth Keebler-Ross. This connection alone made our time together special.

March 10, another *last* came today. We were going to go to dinner with friends. By 4pm both of our energy levels waned and we decided to call and cancel. We ordered pizza.

Breakfast and lunch were still OK, but dinner was now out. John ate his Red Velvet cake and ice cream at 4pm and went to bed to read.

On March 11, we received an authorization for John to reenter pulmonary rehab. I knew Dr. F was thinking curative medicine. He was ordering this so John could retain maximal physical endurance. His heart was in the right place, but why should John drive one hour each way to spend 60 to 90 minutes in lectures and rehab when he had diminishing endurance/energy?

On March 11, two hospice providers visited. Nancy the social worker reviewed and took with her the Advanced Directive copy and contact info so she can assist when John passes on. John was able to tell her that he felt useless and that he could not do anything or help me without collapsing and putting on his oxygen. They discussed these feelings, but this still left John feeling inadequate. This was horrible for a man who had been so dynamic throughout his entire life.

On the same day we also had a visit from Dr. V, a fourth MD.

She was excellent in her history taking assessment and asked John if he ever heard the terms "Congestive heart failure." He turned to me with a questioning look on his face and asked, "Have I?"

I reviewed John's extensive pulmonary/cardiac evals/diagnosis with her, because she did not have the entire medical record. She kindly told John that he had congestive heart failure. She drew the picture of the heart/lungs and their interconnecting functions and how John's body was deteriorating.

When she was done John asked what can be done and she answered the only thing would be a heart and lung transplant, and John was not a candidate. The cut off age is 55. Plus I did not believe that John could withstand and live through such a procedure. Again reality took its toll. He told her what a good life he/ we had, and he was not ready to die. However God was the one in charge. Dr. V reaffirmed.

She then reviewed his meds and said she would make adjustments as time progressed. She agreed that the pulmonary rehab was not a good idea at that time. I would call and cancel that on Monday. We also discussed John's panic attack and anxiety of drowning/ suffocating. She recommended John take ½ an Ativan at night. She also explained to him that there was fluid build-up in his body.

John asked, "Why am I so tired? All I want to do is sleep." Dr. V kindly explained that she had just come from another patient with fibrosis who was bed ridden. Dr. V thought John was doing great compared to what his medical record read. She also told him it was perfectly fine for him to sleep as much as his body wanted and needed. That was reassuring for him.

Two things happened the week of March 13, 2011, that proved how generous others are. Nic had returned from work trips and knew that John was getting worse. She took a look at me and said, "Mom we are trading places this weekend before I return to San Francisco. You need to go to my condo, rest, read, relax, and stop worrying about dad for while I am there."

The next was the hardest. I said, "I don't know if I can do that."

When she asked why, I said that I did not think John's death was imminent, but what if she found her father dead? She responded, "Unfortunately, I now heard you when you said dad has heart failure. I was in denial and did not hear it when you said it before. Mom, I will see dad when he dies, I cannot let you handle this alone, I am here for you, please, let me help."

When did she get so smart?

They had a fun weekend planned anyway – movie and Chinese food. She needed these times for her memory bank. OK, I would go to her condo. Geez, letting go is hard for us stubborn people. I certainly needed the rest. Again I felt so blessed to have her for a daughter.

This week also found me at my primary care physician's office. I had to give in and get an Rx for sleep and for my overactive bladder. Everything gets worse with stress.

Not only that but Dr. R told me it had been two years since I had a physical and - oh joy - she is scheduling a colonoscopy. I knew that I had to take care of myself, so I acquiesced.

During the week of March 13th, John's breathing changed at night. When he was laying on his right side his respirations were gurgling and sounded like he was blowing bubbles. This caused me insomnia as I tried to remember where and when I had last heard that type of breathing.

Linda, nurse case manager, came on March 14 and she verified, "Yes, congestive heart failure." Linda and I reviewed John's meds and organized them. I had reviewed his meds a month previous. I was trying to give John as much independence as possible. Big mistake! Suffice it to say I was glad he did not endanger himself. The meds were now put in a container with four separate doses.

Additionally, Nic told me that I looked and talked like I was exhausted. She adamantly told me that I would be changing places with her the weekend of 3/19. She would bring Molly, her cat, and stay with John. I would go to her place for a much needed respite.

Our daughter, who is a force onto herself and stubborn indeed, told me again that she could not lose both parents; I had to take care of myself. John and Nic would have a good time, see movies and eat Chinese food. When I protested because of John's changed breathing, she asked if I was going to deprive her of quality time with her dad. End of conversation, I would go to her place and I looked forward to the time to regroup/recharge.

We had entered hospice early, or so we thought. It had given us time to know the team and the team to get to know us.

The weekend of 3/19/11 was a special weekend for

John and Nic. They spent entire weekend together. They went to a movie and watched TV. John cherished this weekend. Nic will cherish it for life. Nic told me later that John ran out of oxygen during the movie. They stayed to see the end then she brought him home. He went to bed with the oxygen. John later told me he thought his time of going to movies at a theater were over – another *last*.

He also said that he was going to stop inviting people for visits. He no longer had the energy for it anymore – another *last*. Each last event seemed so final.

My weekend of reading, rest and recharging came to an abrupt halt at 1am on March 20. I had taken the prescribed sleeping pill at 9pm.

About 1am, I had a dream. I saw a gurney and ambulance leaving with a dead person in it. I looked outside. There was no ambulance and everything was quiet. I did not want to call home in case both John and Nic were sleeping. I immediately had the thought that I had to go home. When I got home Nic was still watching TV and attempting to fall asleep. I hugged her and asked if she was OK. She asked why I came home in the middle of the night.

I went to John. He was sleeping, but when I woke him, he also wanted to know why I came home, and then said, "Gee, I'm glad you're home."

"Me also." So much for a planned respite.

March 21

I was on 'total overload' and left my car keys in a jacket twenty-five miles from where I was. Annie had to take me back to get them. I had to ask myself where my brain was these days? MIA, missing in action, I thought.

On 3/26 and 3/27, John had bowel movements with bright red blood. I called both the palliative care nurse and Linda the hospice nurse. None of John's meds contained aspirin. I had discontinued John's aspirin the week before, but it had a 5 day half life, meaning that it takes twice that long for it to be totally out of the body.

He did not have dark, tarry stools, indicative of a bleeding ulcer, so I thought it was probably a hemorrhoid or polyp. The palliative care nurse said we could bring him in to be checked. Yes, of course, but at this stage I am not subjecting him to rectal exams or a colonoscopy. I treated the bleeding with Vaseline to lubricate the rectal area. This was very uncomfortable mentally and physically for John. My assurances that I had seen, cleansed and treated many patients did not appease his discomfort. He was fairly agitated. I increased his Ativan to TID (three times/day).

Our goal was comfort and symptom relief. That was the first promise I made to John when he was diagnosed and would/will remain the focus. Dignity was so important now.

John was sleeping more, partially from the meds but as the hospice doctor told him – that was what his body needed now.

The week of 3/27/11 found us seduced into thinking maybe this disease could be handled with John's cocktail of medications: Vicodin, Ativan, and Viagra three times a day in addition to ones previously that John was taking. Taken regularly John's symptoms of breathlessness, anxiety, and agitation were controlled. On March 30, we met friends in Solana Beach for a great lunch and sharing. It was a beautiful spring day and we had a great time. We did not take John's noon meds with us. After we lunched, we ran errands and returned home at 2pm. Reality set in. John was having labored breathing. He was anxious and short tempered.

~ It is easy to be seduced into thinking things are like they used to be. Of course that is what we want to believe. Our lives had changed and we wanted him symptom free, so we would not leave the house again for several hours without his meds.

Chapter 25

Losing the Battle

April 2 was a very different day at our home. I had planned to walk with friends. When John awakened he seemed quiet. I made him hot chocolate and gave him a donut. He had his book and was sitting in the sun. I asked if he wanted me to cancel my walk; his response was, "Absolutely not." When I returned home John was still in his robe, very unusual for him. I asked if there was anything he wanted to talk about, "No". As the day progressed he watched TV, had lunch, and his Red Velvet cake and ice cream at 4pm. Then said he was going to bed.

I went into the bedroom. He was crying silently sitting on the bed. After some prodding he said he had been trying to out run this disease. This was the reason for his seemingly renewed energy the last few days/weeks. He said, "I pushed myself and thought I could get better and beat this. I have never had anything I could not beat before. But I am losing this battle." I asked him to come out into the living room and sit in his recliner; I gave him another ½ Ativan. We both cried, and I massaged his legs and arms with lavender scented baby oil.

John told me he missed Nic and me already – 42 years had passed so rapidly. He again expressed concerns about what it would feel like to die. Would he just stop breathing? Would he feel as if he was drowning? I asked if he wanted to discuss this with the hospice doctor or nurse. He thought that would help.

John previously had used his sense of humor and avoidance when the hospice workers were here. He said he could only discuss this with me. I had never seen John so clingy/dependent before. He finally said, "I don't want us to cry anymore. We should read and try to get some sleep." The Ativan kicked in and John was able to sleep, but his respirations had changed. He had long pauses between breaths. I asked myself, "Is this the function of the Vicodin or disease progression?" I didn't like the answer to this question. Before John fell asleep he again took me to his computer and reviewed our finances and all bank accounts and expenditures.

My brother Johnny was scheduled to visit us on April 7. I asked if John wanted me to cancel the visit. His response was, "No."

I despised the feelings of finality that I was experiencing. John asked, "You will miss me?"

God yes I would miss him.

Later when he was sleeping I went to the kitchen to get a glass of water. When I returned he asked, "Who is here, your lover?" I wanted to scream, where in the hell is that coming from? But instead, I hugged him and told him he was my lover.

Millions did this every day, why did I feel so helpless? We both knew we had no control over the disease, and that we had done everything we could do. Together we would transition this passage. But I did not know how yet.

April 3

Caregivers are not angels. We have our breaking points. Dottie, my RN friend for 30 years told me a few weeks previous that I might experience angry feelings with John. I assured her I got over my anger, Yah right!!!!!!

John had and an especially bad day yesterday: remorseful, crying, concerned that Nic and I would forget him, and anxious with more questions. How he would feel when he died, would he feel like he is drowning and not able to get his breath. We talked, cried, hugged and I gave him ½ Ativan, massaged him with lavender mineral oil.

He went to sleep. I on the other hand was restless, listening to his moist breathing and irregular respiratory pattern. To say I was sleep deprived on this night was an understatement. Additionally, this was my prep day for a colonoscopy tomorrow. Not a pleasant experience. John was able to go to the Jacuzzi. He was gone a long time, so I went to check on him.

He was quiet, withdrawn and when I asked him if he wanted to talk about anything – yes he said. He has been thinking about all of his friends in Des Moines to whom he had not said goodbye. John was the best person that I have known to keep in contact with his friends. He talked and reminisced continually, so I didn't get it.

He wanted to make a CD of his life, then, after he died, he wanted me to take the CD to Des Moines and have a reminiscing party with his friends – half of whom I did not know.

I would not lie to him, but was angry that he would expect that.

We decided against that idea. We would celebrate his life here. We would not have a service afterwards because his body was being donated to UCSD for research. Since January we had nonstop family and friends here.

I believe in giving 110% while people live — then live with their spirit and accept what cannot be changed. I had no clue what that would look like. I knew for sure that I would do anything for John, but did not think that I would have the energy to 'party' with his friends.

Nic visited. They went to lunch and after they re-turned we all discussed John's wishes again. We agreed that he would make the CD and send money to his friend to have a gathering to watch the CD, and reminisce the "good, bad and ugly." (His words, not mine).

I guess my exhaustion and anger boiled over. Care-givers aren't saints and we have our limits.

The good news was that my mammogram and co-lonoscopy were normal. Thank you God.

April 6

Another hospice nurse visited. John discussed a recent panic attack. The nurse said it was time to start using Morphine for *air hunger*. When she said *air hunger* John immediately responded, "That is exactly what it feels like when I can't get my breath." She also recommended increasing the Ativan 1 TID and liberal use of meds. Substitute Morphine for Vicodin.

We also chose to have the primary care physician switched to the hospice physician. This team worked great together and we had confidence that this is the greatest quality of care, empathy, and compassion. This stage needed to preserve John's dignity. Pat, the hospice Chaplin, and my brother Johnny would visit the next day. John was at peace with these decisions and peacefully sleeping.

I got the feeling he was crossing off a list of things he needed to make sure happen before he died. His anxiety had diminished and he was comfortable.

April 7

Pat the spiritual advisor visited. Along with her spiritual message she imparted the fact that caregiver family members who are in healthcare have a difficult time relinquishing that role, i.e., it was time for me to be a wife, not a nurse. Whoa – did she have a magnifying glass into my brain?

Additionally, she intuited that my resistance for starting John on Morphine was the ingrained fact that I saw Morphine as a respiratory depressant.

She reminded me that John was getting a very small dose of morphine and that he was a big guy; therefore he could withstand this amount of morphine to control his anxious respiratory symptoms and fear of drowning. Geez, my control issue again. Anyway, her advice proved to be right on.

With the increased Ativan and Morphine, John was relaxed and breathing easier. John took a long nap before Johnny arrived, we had lunch and they decided to have another trip to the casino, my least favorite place in the world. But I was doing what John wanted to do these days. The results were a fun afternoon with John being a big winner. He would split the money with Nic for her new floors. The observers advised John he would receive a 1099 for taxes. Yah, I would have to deal with that next year.

~ I had a sign on my desk reminding me to be open and receptive to all good. Part of that is accepting the advice from the hospice team, giving up the control, relaxing, and being grateful as I hear John's relaxed breathing as he sleeps. I learned something new every day. Joy!!!

Chapter 26

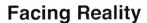

Facing Reality

Week of April 11

Nic was staying with us for 5 days. Nic had been very stoic but finally allowed herself to see the reality of what was happening to John. She cried and sobbed that she did not know how she would live without her father. He had always been there for her.

As parents we had been criticized of being too protective of Nic. I disagreed, of course. She and I talked, cried and planned how we would cope after John's death.

This probably sounds weird, but as previously stated, I believe in giving 110% while my loved ones are living. We cannot change the course of John's *rhythm of life disease,* we can only control how we respond and react to it.

We agreed that we had celebrated John's/our life and we would find a way to cope. We did things differently in this family. Nic asked if we could go to her place to hibernate, mourn, veg, sleep, cry, and talk for a few days after we take care of the vital things after John died. As I saw it, that was a wonderful plan. Everyone had been terrific – family, friends, visiting non-stop with food, plants, and flowers, sharing, caring with so much love; but we were exhausted.

Nic and I decided we are introverts. No one would guess that about either of us because of the jobs we have done entertaining, but we both know we value our alone time and would need that to heal. After things were taken care of, Nic and I planned to go on a trip.

We had friends visit for lunch on Sunday and Wednesday. I withheld John's meds on Sunday. He did not do well that night. I was learning and attempting to adapt with each change in John. He was absolutely an extrovert and wanted people around, and then he would collapse. His recuperative time was longer after each visit now. How long could we continue to do this?

Nic had her taxes done on April 12th. She was thrilled that she had a refund. She came home ecstatic and wanted to take us to dinner. John declined stating he did not have the energy, but he wanted us to go.

I gave him his meds, left him another Ativan to take if he started to feel anxious. We went to the beach and had a great dinner, talked and were relaxed for the first time in who knows how long. When we got home John was anxious, had a barky like cough and air hunger. Damn!!!

I gave him lots of meds, he finally was able to sleep (not fitfully) we were up three times getting more meds. In the morning I called Linda, the hospice nurse. She recommended the nebulizer treatment to see if that would relieve John's symptoms. She also asked if I wanted a hospital bed delivered. I didn't think we needed that yet, but the question re-enforced that where we were in the battle. I was able to give John the meds through his C-pap, but needed an in-service on the correct use of the nebu-lizer.

John's response to all of this was that he would try to make jokes and tell me I that was too serious. The joking aggravated me and I had difficulty han-dling it. I did not see the humor in any of this. I attributed it to, "Men are from Mars, Women are from Venus." I just didn't get it.

John also repeatedly questioned every hospice worker asking if they thought his fibrosis was caused from the asbestos exposure and why his claim wasn't accepted yet. His main concern was that I would get some of his retirement when he died. He was obsessed with this and had made nu-merous calls to the VA who were adjudicating the case.

On April 13, the hospice team discussed John's case. Resulting phone calls were: a person would come and review the nebulizer usage and a social worker would attempt to contact the VA regarding John's claim. They requested that I resend the por-tion of the VA disability findings of asbestos expo-sure and pleural plaque in 1992 and 1996. John had not had time to develop asbestosis/fibrosis by then. It takes 25-35 years for the symptoms to develop. This was all submitted in the package in January, but I would resubmit it. The hospice doctor also recommended revisiting the possibility of a lung biopsy and second opinion. Again, I was not willing to shorten John's life and take the risk of a lung biopsy for money.

John was sleeping comfortably after the nebulizer treatment.

Oxygen was delivered and the nebulizer procedure was reviewed, which was added to John's treatment plan.

The nebulizer treatment did not relieve John's symptoms and the barky cough. John had asked Linda, the RN, the day before if the meds he was taking would extend his life. She reaffirmed that we were looking for quality, not quantity of life.

I had tried lemon cough drops, honey and eucalyptus, none of which relieved John's cough. Another call to the triage hospice nurse who said she could call in an order to the pharmacy. I would have to pick this up. John was on the phone and said he did not want me to leave. Earlier in the day he said, "Please don't leave me." So I increased John's morphine and another Ativan and he was able to sleep fitfully. When Linda called me she asked if I wanted the hospital bed delivered. Reality is everywhere, every conversation. No were not ready for the hospital bed.

April 14

I moved furniture so we would eventually be able to move the bed into John's office. That is where his TV and computer were. We added Netflix and John's favorite music to the computer, so this was where he would be most comfortable. I would move a futon into the room for me to sleep when the next stage comes, which was way sooner than we were mentally ready for.

God this is hard!!!

Nic had been here the week of April 11th. She went home on April 15th. John became very anxious with air hunger and walked to the patio to see if he could breathe easier. He was talking like he thought this was the end of his life. I called Nic back. We sat on the futon on the patio, hugged, cried, talked.

I had done a nebulizer treatment when his cough started.

It is a vicious cycle when the *anxiety-air hunger cycle starts.* I had given him Ativan, morphine and robitusin with codeine. He still was not calming down. After increasing the morphine I called the hospice nurse. She advised I was doing everything right, but to increase the morphine to 20mgs every 2 hours, if needed. Finally, he was able to rest. Saturday morning John slept late. When he awakened, he asked if it was nice out, he wanted to go to the Jacuzzi. Nic and I helped him to the Jacuzzi. It was a glorious sunny day and he loved it. Another *last* I thought.

I called several family members and friends who were still planning to come and advised them John was not up to guests. People could not believe they were getting this call. This was not the "vivacious, fun loving, gregarious John." Sorry, but true.

After the Jacuzzi, an oxygen rest and more meds he was able to eat some of the lunch. He asked, "I am failing fast, right?"

John was unsteady on his feet. He was trying to brush his teeth and fell in the bathroom. It was hard to not hover and try and let him be independent, but try to keep him safe.

John deleted two things from his 'to do list'. He helped Nic return her car and finalize the lease return agreement. And we received notification that the VA has accepted his claim for 'asbestosis/fibrosis'.

Sunday morning John got up to go to the bathroom. I asked him to stay there while I went to the other bathroom and that he should "wait until I get back." He was so funny these days. He always had an incredible sense of humor - his defense mechanism.

He asked why I "wanted to get a three year old cat."

Nic had to maintain as much normalcy (whatever that is) as possible, so I encouraged her to return to work. It would give her a much needed break from the constant stress of watching her dad deteriorate. I convinced her that we all loved each other very much, and if she did not see her dad takes his last breath it would be OK. She finally acquiesced.

Surviving Caregiving

Chapter 27

The Final Days

April 19

Nic called from San Francisco. John had fallen 5 times last night. He was disoriented, aggressive, and angry because he couldn't get comfortable.

The *air hunger* followed by anxiety is a cycle that is horrific to watch. I called Linda the hospice nurse at 6am expecting to get her voicemail. She picked up and started the process by ordering a hospital bed. Crisis care was started at 9:30am with continuous critical care. My God, how do people go through this without hospice? Nic returned home from San Francisco to the worst nights of our lives.

John's anxiety was uncontrollable, even though he had enough meds to make most people sleep for weeks. John paced the floor, while leaning backwards and falling if 2 people were not supporting him. He had become aggressively delusional and paranoid.

He constantly asked Nic and I if we were killing him. Then he asked if he had killed someone.

He was crawling over the hospital bedside rails. Nic and I moved a futon close to the bed. We laid on the futon and tried to soothe John and keep him from panicking. His symptoms progressed. Hospice tried to decide whether the anxiety was from infection or if he was actively dying.

A friend called that night from Des Moines. I told him it was too late to visit. John heard me and said, "So this is it?"

I replied, "Yes, you have done everything for Nic and me, and it is time for you to be at peace."

Nic and I released John telling him that we did not want him to suffer anymore. He said, "It's too bad they can't give me something." We agreed.

Dr. Kevorkian should be sainted.

John's cough was unmanageable – he could not cough up asbestos. Our strong viable, courageous, protective father/husband could not beat this horrible disease.

John had all of his meds, he was sitting on the sofa with Nic massaging his shoulders and hugging him.

Family, friends, hospice, and the VA palliative nurse all called to offer respite options. The whole world had been so wonderful. We did feel blessed.

April 21

John, heavily medicated and pacing the floor, walked up to the Nurse Practitioner, who was in the process of trying to figure what she could do to make him more peaceful, winked and said, "Wanna dance honey?"

The people at the table lost it, how could he be so humorous while so medicated, and so agitated all at the same time. No one knew that answer, but it would help Nic and I to remember the humorous parts of all of this week.

If I wrote the amount of meds that he had in his body, you would question my sanity and call me a liar, saying that it was impossible. Prior to that night I felt the same way. We had a male nurse that night. About midnight he called Nic and I who had just lain down. John had become even more aggressive, combative, swinging at us. He forced his way out of the front door with three of us trying to hold him back. Thank God it was 2:30 AM because he was only wearing his boxers. Finally, we convinced him to return to the house. He had called 911 twice. Nic managed to call the police and tell them the situation.

The hospice nurse called for backup. He was advised that the current situation was too out of control and we needed to call EMT's to take him to the hospital. By policy in our area, ambulances will only transport 25 miles. The VA Palliative Care Unit was 28 miles away. The nurse, Nic, and I worked together to get John in the car. It was no easy job, but we managed to get him to the ER.

The amount of Ativan if took to get John under control was enormous. One male provider quietly kept telling John not pull on the bedside rails and that he could hurt himself. John would reply, "Yes sir." Then within seconds he would scream swearing to let him out. The providers were great and I left a message for Michael, the palliative care nurse case manager. I told him that we were in ER and in need of a bed. He worked his magic and John was transferred to that unit. Again this unit was absolutely amazing.

The team evaluated John, and medications were administered. John was incredibly strong and was fighting sleep. We believed he was afraid to go to sleep thinking that he would not wake up. Nic and I both released him from this world. We could not fathom how we would survive without John but we also did not want to see him suffer, mentally or physically.

My family made sure that John was saved and going to Heaven. I never doubted this. John had been a wonderful father, husband, and provider. The disease turned him into someone we did not know. We ached seeing him like this and breathing so harshly.

Nic and I went to her home to get some rest and feed Molly the cat. Nic had bad dreams and very restless sleep. I could not sleep and returned to the hospital. John had hit two hospital employees. Thank God they were not seriously injured.

Words cannot describe John's combative behavior. Again this was not the person we loved. The kind, gentle, loving person we knew was MIA (missing in action). Nic had brought my lavender oil and some vitamin E oil. Once John was medicated appropriately and finally resting for the first time in a week, I massaged his feet, hands, and arms with lavender and vitamin E oil. The room was filled with the calming aroma.

Surviving Caregiving

Chapter 28

The Long Struggle is Finally Over

April 23

This was officially the worst night of our lives. Nic and I massaged John, hugged, kissed and released him. John died as he lived. He kept his sense of humor and fought for life. His body defied all odds and he died at 5 AM.

Surviving Caregiving

Chapter 29

Remembering Our John

John never met a stranger and kept in contact with people that he had known for 60 plus years. They all thought John was the hilarious and carefree. John loved life and people but he was haunted from a dysfunctional childhood. It was no one's fault. Lengthy parental illnesses robbed him of the love and home that all children deserve. John's childhood tormented him. As he died, the rage we witnessed seemed to be him wrestling with inner torment.

It was horrible to watch the progression of John's disease. He did not look sick, in fact he had lost weight and people frequently commented that he looked better than he had in years. He did, but this disease was an insidious killer of John's lungs and heart.

Most people that we contacted about John's death were literally shocked because he minimized his symptoms, remained active and we celebrated his life. John used humor and sarcasm to keep the darker feelings at bay – dread, uncertainty, abject fear, and regret. I had never once seen John fearful in 42+ years. A song comes to mind that epitomizes the John most people knew, *The clown laughing on the outside and crying on the inside.*

Air hunger caused horrific physiological, mental, physical pain. No matter how much medication he had, nothing touched the air hunger.

John was the best provider, husband, and father. He knew his end was coming soon. We honestly talked about it frequently. John trusted Nic and me to always be truthful with him. As hard as that was, it had to be.

Our family values encompass love, truth and honesty, even if it is painful. But we had promised John *respect and dignity,* and we had to keep these as our focus to see us through this storm.

Nic and I were numb, mentally and physically exhausted. We went back to her home and were dealing as best we could. We had lost the love of our life, but we vowed to live on with John's spirit at the core of our hearts. I wished Nic did not have to experience the last week of John's life but our family takes care of each other and so we were a team to the end. The tsunami had passed.

We knew our hearts are strong organs. We could be mad that John was not physically with us. However, that would not cover our sadness. We knew the best way to love John was to let him go. Our grief would have a pace of its own. The only thing we knew for sure was that we were strong, stubborn women and we would survive.

Nic and I wanted the compassionate dignified death that John deserved. The John we saw the last week was not the person we loved for 40 plus years. I never wanted Nic to hear John's *death rattle*. You only have to hear it once for it to bring nightmares for life. The palliative care staff liberally medicated John so it lasted only a few hours, but what horrendous hours.

John's last four hours were peaceful. Because of John's agitation, he had 24-hour observation. The kindest, sweetest, loving visitor was with us Friday night. I did not even know his last name, but would find out later because he needed to know how grateful we were for his kindness. Nic and I kissed John numerous times and told him we loved him and that he could go in peace.

At one point when Nic kissed John, he opened his eyes and they shined with pure love. The attendant was the first to tell Nic about this. He made sure Nic knew. I prayed that it would ease the horrific pain we experienced.

April 27

John's decision to live life to the fullest and not have a service after his death left a void for family and friends. Nic and I were overwhelmed with the love, food, plants, from family and friends. They wanted to have a party to celebrate John's life.

Remember – John was the extrovert, me, the introvert, could not handle a party at this point. Sleep had evaded both Nic and I. She had nightmares of the *death rattle*. My manic nature pushed me to tear the house apart, removing hospice supplies and all images of John's disease and hellish *end of life*. As you will read later I totally believe in Feng Shui, and wanted to return our home to a healthy, happy, harmonious space. Staying in tuned to Nic's needs were my priorities.

Other people's grief could be dealt with later. I agreed to discuss a party after we recooperated, slept, dealt with legal matters. Nic and I would take a healing trip, and then maybe I could consider a party at the pool. John loved the pool, but I did not know if I could do that. Only time would tell. This present time was about Nic and I handling our grief. Only we could know what would work best for us.

Chapter 30

Our Life Without John

April 29 was a horrible day. I finally hit my wall. I had no energy and could not imagine getting dressed. Bob Sharp, the man who introduced John and I forty-three years ago, came the day before. It took all of my energy to visit with Bob and his family. Nic and I went to dinner. Sleep was difficult these days. John slept with a C-pap for 15 years before his diagnosis, then had the noisier concentrator, so I was used to those noises. I kept waking up, listening and not hearing them and thinking something had happened to John, and then I remembered. I read letters and cards.

The cards from Larry Young and Adam hit me and I started to cry. My brother Johnny and Charlene were scheduled to visit. I did not think that I had the energy to get dressed and called Johnny to ask him not to come. He listened, but said that I needed family, and they were coming. It didn't matter if I got dressed or not. I kept hearing John's horrible last words to me when I would not have his restraints removed.

He swore, called me horrible names and said I was finally getting what I wanted. Nic was not there and I had not told her this yet. What if that is what John actually thought? The tears had finally come. I called Nic and she was on her way. Pat, the hospice Chaplin called to say the hospice team did not think John's anxiety was spiritual. I concurred. John knew he was saved and going to heaven. The falls, his head injury, air hunger, PTSD all combined to make John's last days so horrific.

April 29

Johnny and Charlene arrived and I was still in my robe. They thought going out for Mexican food and margaritas would help me, so I got dressed and we left. It did help. Johnny later told me when I called, all he could think of was Rick, our brother who committed suicide. I was definitely sad, and crying for John BUT NEVER, NEVER SUICIDAL.

When a family has a history of suicide by one of its members, the thought of suicide pops into our minds when another member is depressed.

Nic, Johnny, Charlene and I talked about John's last days. The next morning Johnny and I walked three miles. He told me I was walking slower than the last time we walked. No Shit. My energy was depleted, I had gained weight and I was numb, as was Nic. I knew it would take time.

May 4

Reality kept hitting me in the face. I had gone to run errands and get my haircut. I had dealt with another insurance issue and was late, forgot my cell phone. I was gone 4 hours before I realized I did not have my cell. When I came home Nic was calling in a panic about where I had been. I had a coughing spell the last night she stayed with us and she was panicked that she was going to lose me also, and then she would be all alone. Wow, we kept having these "mini melt downs."

Normal, I knew, but not the normal for us previously.

Then the death certificates arrived. Another whole *land mine*, dealing with the legal issues started in earnest. I think we were both numb. How long would this pain last?

Surviving Caregiving

Chapter 31

End of Life Legal Details

In the days after John's passing, we received so many phone calls, cards, food, love, and hugs that we were overwhelmed.

Next we would need to deal with all the end of life legal aspects.

This task is incredibly gut wrenching. I had to repeat the same thing so many times that I was on autopilot. Why isn't there a central clearinghouse for reporting and dealing with this process?

Here are a few of the legal details for immediate concern:

- You must produce a death certificate or confirmation of death within 14 days to receive your benefits

- Expect at least 40 minutes with Social Security for taped interview

- For "Loss of Life and Gap insurance." ADVICE: READ THE FINE PRINT. This will probably be when you are stressed with dealing with a loved one's illnesses issues. As of writing this, I do not have a final decision yet, but how uncouth of John for dying three days before the six-month waiting period to collect on this policy. And this was recommended by a trusted friend at our bank, of course she had no way of knowing when John would die

My frustration was off the charts. However there had been kind cooperative people to help me traverse this situation. UCSD body donor spokes person gave me tremendous advice early today. She told me to ignore all advice people gave me at this time.

She said 99.9% of the advice will be incorrect, but easily by well-meaning people and other people's experience would not be mine.

May 6 found me processing more insurance forms. When I tried to access John's credit union account online, which I am a joint member, I was locked out and needed to call Decedent Affairs. After review they reopened the account so I could access it. Yes headquarters received the death certificate and application for *loss of life* insurance, which we bought.

It was under review, but John died before the six month waiting period, so the representative said the claim would not be paid. READ THE FINE PRINT, EVEN IF YOU ARE STRESSED TO THE MAX. The term of that policy was not primary on my mind during the last week of John's life. Nic's and my survival and attempting to cope with the situation took more energy than either of us had. We were still in shock and numb.

John's psychiatrist called after hearing about John's aggressive anger and rage. He agreed that the air hunger along with probable head traumas and medications were contributing factors, but he thought John's PTSD was the most likely cause of the rage. He assured me the last session he had with John was positive. John said he knew he was going to die but had to make sure everything was taken care of for Nic and I first. He also knew John well enough to know John would never intentionally hurt us. Reassuring, yes, but it was difficult to forget that last week. The psychiatrist recommended Nic and I take advantage of the bereavement resources available to us.

May 8

Our year of *firsts* begins. On Mother's Day, Nic and I went to a movie and lunch. If Mother's day were this difficult without John, what would Thanksgiving and Christmas be like?

May 9

Endurance, patience and perseverance were needed to wade through the voluminous paperwork that needed to be done. I thought I was prepared by having all contacts, phone numbers, and agencies filed in our trust book. This process would have been worse if I actually had to gather all of that after John's death. Even having the above did not make this process easy.

If you have a trust everything needs to be notarized. Most banks no longer have notaries, but UPS does. Banks need to modify trust forms to ensure Nic followed me in the trust order. We thought that was already done, but the banks had changed policies/forms in the year since we finalized the trust.

I knew the trip to the VA Hospital would be traumatic. I had taken John there so many times over the last year, but today I was making the trip alone to hand in the DIC (Dependency and Compensation) forms to apply for benefits from John's "asbestosis and pulmonary fibrosis caused by his asbestos exposure from *rip outs* on Navy ships without respiratory protection."

This would take more weeks/months to be adjudicated. I called to check if I needed anything except the form to be completed and was told, "No". I should have known better. Even though the computer gave the person all of John's dates of service and retirement info, I had to submit a DD214.

Next I went to the Palliative Care Unit. I again wanted to compliment them on the care John received. Yes, it is their job, but this staff did not *just do their jobs*. John's treatment under the worst of conditions, with his combativeness and agitation, made me proud to be in the health care system.

The VA gets a bad rap. It is true that access is a problem. They are overwhelmed with people returning from combat. They are under staffed and probably under paid. I do not compliment healthcare lightly. After 40 plus years as a nurse I truly value what this staff did for John and our family. There are not sufficient adjectives to express Nic's and my gratitude. The check I gave them, and a letter of appreciation would have to do. I was still considering volunteering to do foot, hand reflexology for staff members and the caregivers. The focus would be on the patient and family – where it should be.

The stress of the staff and caregivers is expected, but not addressed. Time would tell how I would give back. I first needed to complete the voluminous paperwork, go to Iowa with Johnny and check on family members who were not healthy. Next Nic and I would take our healing trip, and then I would decide what would come next.

The day ended by taking the notarized form to the insurance company to process the life insurance. I thought the federal government was bad for paperwork. Insurance companies may run a close second.

Nic was trying to be good to herself and started a Yoga class. It had been too long since she was able to focus on her health. I was so happy that she had begun that process.

May 11

What a terrific day. I felt guilty writing that so soon after John's death. I started out by touching up some of the walls that had marks from John's falls and other neglected areas in our home. This led to some creative painting of picture frames and other things.

I thought that it was nice that no one was yelling at me telling me I should not be breathing paint fumes. Then I caught myself, should I actually feel this, yes I do and it is OK. John was a great guy, but very controlling. Shocker, huh?

UPS brought the insurance check and two hours were spent at the credit union paying off the house and car. Nic joined me for lunch. She is thrilled for me.

Dr. F called. This call truly surprised me. We were fairly certain he hated us after our first meeting. He grew on us and apparently we grew on him also. He expressed his condolences, asked about Nic and me. I told him that I was writing this book and he had to tell me now if he did not want to be a part of it.

Surprised yet again, not only that but he would like to read about our experiences to see if it might help him understand patient's with pulmonary fibrosis. I told him I might volunteer with reflexology at the VA for healthcare providers and caregivers. He not only encouraged this but also asked me to stop and see him at the VA. He provided his email address. He admitted that he had never seen a family like ours and also said that our daughter would fight (maybe not the right word) for her father.

They loved each other very much. All true and she did fight for him. They were each other's constant cheerleaders. When I called Nic she was equally surprised and agreed the phone call was nice. It felt good to have a good day.

On May 12, I awakened with a sore throat and laryngitis. I had been going on reserve the last few/weeks/months and finally my body said enough. After making my ginger tea concoction and inhaling eucalyptus I finally decided I needed a down day. As Rosemary says, "The body rules." Unlike other times in my life, I did not push myself. It felt good to be able to breathe and take care of myself.

Nic continued her daily Yoga. I prayed we were on our road to recovery. Again, we needed to be good to ourselves, guilt free.

John is imprinted on our brains, but now we must find our new paths with his wonderful spirit as our guide. I always had a purpose in life and a zillion things to be done. This day seemed strange. It was quiet, so unusual. I had always cherished "peace, quiet, and tranquility" but this was still a tremendous adjustment.

May 14

Nic and Molly the cat came to spend the weekend. We were going to a surprise luncheon for a friend who was receiving a presidential citation for her work with the Military Officer's Association of American – MOAA. It seemed like a fun event.

Well, yes, it would have been except the guest speaker was the widower of a Naval Admiral speaking about Department of Defense and how Congress is passing bills to cut the budget by re- fusing to pay "widower benefits for servicemen/women who died of service connected disabilities."

Crap, John spent his last few months fighting for

me to receive compensation for his death from asbestosis. An innocent luncheon celebration should have been fun, but we keep getting hit in the face with reality. We were in a crowded room; Nic and I became overcome with sadness and looked for an escape route. We did not want to put a damper on Paulette's awards but could not stay to hear the rest of this presentation.

The real reality is that we would be doing OK, then something would remind us of John. Three weeks is such a short time. Our loss was too raw.

I guessed that this is what surviving the loss of a loved one is all about.

We came home to find a check for $3,600.00 made out to me from the US Treasury in Austin Texas. There was no letter accompanying it, so I do not know what it is for, but had been warned in my hours of phone calls in the last three weeks that it was too late to stop automatic payments to John, so I would have to pay any monies received back to the government. I would deposit the check but not spend it. We thought surely John's life was worth more than $3600, wasn't it? More questions than answers this day, and each question added to our confusion.

Nic and I were missing John terribly. Nic wishes for just one more phone call from dad. She did not know how she would live without him. He was the measuring stick for all relationships and was always our fierce protector. We knew we had to fill our lives with more than grief and worry. Hopefully, time would decrease the emotional pain.

The other positive thing that had happened was Molly the cat had returned to her sweet, playful self and was no longer hanging out on top of the kitchen cupboards. Pets must be incredibly sensitive. She knew John was sick. All of the people coming and going disturbed her tranquil environment. We were happy to have her fun loving kitty self back.

May 16

Painters arrived to paint the walls that were damaged by John's falls. But painting is like cleaning, when you do one area, then the rest of the house needs it, so it progressed. It amazed me that friends had an opinion about me having the house painted so soon. They thought that I was not honoring John, I guess. But, I could not have the constant reminders of that horrific last week of John's life.

Our home is our paradise. John's spirit is everywhere. The walls are covered with collages of the fun and wonderful, cherished family vacations. We honor John's spirit by returning our home to the Moody Paradise it was, before John's disease consumed us.

Surviving Caregiving

Chapter 32

Life, Force, Spirit

John found acceptance long before Nic and I did. In Sept 2010 he said, "I feel better, I'm not depressed anymore. I know you don't want to hear it, but I really have turned it over to the man upstairs – God."

John had a *to do* list and was able to check off the last two items on the last lucid day of his life - April 15th. I believe people keep themselves alive long enough to take care vital business. If John did accept his finality, he sure as heck fought hard the last week of his life to let us know he was still the fighter we knew and loved.

Writing this journal was therapeutic for me. I have always believed in journaling to help work through and resolve issues.

I feel calmer and know we will take everything as it comes, and deal with it as we Moody's always have. We have a saying in our family *–Yea for us.* It gives us strength.

John read the first pages of this book and said to me, "Our life has not been sad. This book should be about 42 years of togetherness. Why all the sadness? You have to expand this."

I realized that he was right and began including the joyful times of our journey together in this missive. Collaborating with my husband in this creation process became a sharing, caring experience.

Where to go from here? I learned a long time ago when something disastrous happens, something good usually follows it. This time I wanted to let it develop. I wanted to try and go with the flow.

I know I will find my next purpose in life. I will try and be open and receptive to all good. I believe each person is responsible for our own health, happiness, and harmony. We are trying to concentrate on our mental, physical, spiritual wellbeing. I know Nic and I are stubborn enough to find our own paths. Helen Keller said, "When one door closes, a window opens." I want my window to show me peace, tranquility and serenity.

John died as he lived. He fought every step of the way. His life force spirit lives on in our hearts and homes.

Addendums

Please note that these suggestions are not meant to usurp legal or medical advice.

Surviving Caregiving

Addendum 1

Homeopathic Remedies for Caregivers

Caregivers are subject to higher stress levels, illnesses (chronic or acute) more frequently then others.

Why? We put others first so we don't take care of ourselves.

Some of my other favorite homeopathic remedies are:

- Ginger tea is very effective for headache and laryngitis. Boil the ginger then add cayenne pepper, cinnamon and honey and drink quarts of it. According to homeopathic literature, ginger raises your body temperature, which helps you fight off viruses. Ginger also has anti-inflammatory and immune supporting properties, which boosts your body's defenses against diseases

- Eucalyptus oil for your sinuses, nose, and throat. Does this remind you of your grandmother's *Vicks* remedies? Vicks has eucalyptus in it. If you don't have access to a sauna, take a hot tub bath, boil water and add eucalyptus, then cover your head and inhale it. If you don't have eucalyptus, use Vicks. Also put Vicks on your feet with warm socks. You will immediately taste the Vicks and it will circulate through your body releasing the toxins. After the sauna, massage your body with sweet almond oil

- Combine a cucumber, lavender oil, and eucalyptus oil in a blender and put it on your face and neck. It is so revitalizing

- Tangerine oil for energy

- Peppermint oil for respiratory inflammation, GI gas, cramps, indigestion. It is also cooling and soothing

- Use Lavender oil for relaxation

- Use above mentioned oils for therapeutic foot & hand reflexology. Reflexology is a great way to stimulate the acupressure points and increases the flow of positive Chi' through the body

- Tub soaks of Epsom salts and oils are revitalizing. I have several oils by my tub and use whichever one I need: lavender, eucalyptus, peppermint, tea tree, rosemary and tangerine. They are so therapeutic. Create your own spa and indulge. You and everyone around you are happier if you are healthy and relaxed

- Fresh vegetable juice is so nourishing and especially needed when stress levels are increased. I use a Vita Mixer because I want the pulp/fiber for my digestive system. But if you have an active digestive system you may want to use a juicer, which removes the pulp. My juice combination is: ginger (fresh), celery, carrots, cucumbers, cabbage, parsley, and beets. Nutritionists will tell you to make this daily. I make enough for a week. If you leave the pulp in you will have to add water so you can drink it

Fresh apple and ginger juice is another of my favorites.

Natural Health magazine recommends, "Juicing vegetables and drinking your homemade concoction is like an IV infusion of the vitamins and minerals your brain needs to function well."

- Turkey noodle soup is a favorite remedy of old. No one really knows why chicken or turkey soup works when your immune system is depleted. Some think it is the potassium. Quite frankly today I don't care why it works, but for me it does. Mind over matter, maybe

- It is a well-known fact that antibiotics will not treat virus infections. The over use of antibiotics makes your body drug resistant, so if you need antibiotics for a serious illness in future, they may not be effective. Additionally, colds normally last 10-14 days with or without antibiotics, so why subject your body to them? I'll bet my remedies will be faster

- Garlic has anti-bacterial properties that also prevent respiratory symptoms from progressing. Cook with it or mix it with honey to eat it raw

The above are combinations homeopathic remedies and common sense. If these remedies help you, great, if not, please seek medical advice. Additional homeopathic remedies and thoughts for our sanity, health, and to purify and detox emotions are listed below. Again, none of these are meant to usurp medical treatment.

- Cucumbers for the eyes are a must for people who cry or do a lot of computer work, studying, and reading. Slice and freeze them, place them over your eyes. They will startle you when they are cold but are soothing and revitalizing

- Sliced lemons and cucumber water are cooling, revitalizing, refreshing, and detoxifying

- A teaspoon of vinegar daily to lower cholesterol levels. Be sure to dilute the vinegar in water. Drinking straight vinegar can cause damage to your throat and esophagus

- Foot soaks of lavender oil, and Epsom salts

- Use clove oil to relieve cold sores. If you put it on when you first feel the burning, it interrupts progression of the blisters and agony. Yes, you will smell like cloves, but for me it is worth it

- Brush your teeth with baking soda to whiten your teeth

- Gliders, rocking chairs are also soothing – if they work for babies, then why not adults?

- Finally, I wash all of my vegetables and fruits in 1/4-cup peroxide in a sink filled with water. I let them set for 5-10 minutes to kill any salmonella. I do this even if the package says they are washed and ready to eat. No one wants salmonella, and I find this is great to kill all bacteria

Surviving Caregiving

Addendum 2

Locus of My Focus – Personal Mantra

Locus of my focus –several times a day, my mantra is, "Thank you God and the universe for my mental, physical, spiritual, financial, and intellectual health, happiness, harmony, peace, tranquility and serenity. I see clearly and am walking on Tamarack beach at age 150."

These are what are important to me – yours will be different. Again our *self-talk*, or mantras, are vitally important to reaffirm what core values we believe in and want for ourselves. Serenity comes from knowing what you can and cannot change. I could not change John's medical condition. But I could change how I reacted to it.

The Serenity prayer says it all. "God grant me the serenity to accept the things I cannot change, the courage to change the things I can, and the wisdom to know the difference." I have this prayer posted several places through our home.

Surviving Caregiving

Addendum 3

Home Sweet Home – Benefits of Feng Shui

Here are a few questions to ask yourself:

Does your Home environment nourish you? Is it your paradise?

Our environment subconsciously influences us so much. Feng Shui is the Chinese art of placement and Chi' energy flow to balance your environment. Whether you believe in this concept or not, take note of how you feel when you enter your home and office spaces. Do you smile or take a huge nourishing breath? Are you inspired? Are you sick a lot, have low energy, and feel like you are in a rut?

It is vital for our health, happiness and harmony, energy and balance that our environment nourishes us. Vital energies (Chi') flow through us connecting us to our environments. Sometimes we develop scotomas – blind spots, and think we have no control over our surroundings. Sometimes this is necessary for financial reasons, but please do not let this become long lasting. It will affect your health and energy.

Feng Shui changes do not need to be expensive.

The colors we live with are so important. Paint is cheap. Have fun with a "make over" and see how you feel when you enter the space afterwards. DO

YOU SMILE?

Light nourishes us and stimulates our serotonin. Open the drapes and let in the natural light.

Add some plants and flowers. Who doesn't feel better when plants live around us?

Harmonious sounds stimulate the positive Chi'. Examples include: fountains, chimes, music, birds, bring in nature.

Aromas nourish and invigorate.

Love your furniture. Avoid sharp corners. Ergonomics at home and in the workplace are important to maintain a pain and injury free environment.

De-clutter, minimize, and recycle what you haven't used or worn in the last 6 mos. When you are organized your stress is reduced, and you easily find what you need. Others will benefit from your recycled treasures.

Detoxify. There are many examples on the Internet. Choose the one that makes the most sense to you.

A Chinese proverb says to move "27 things when you want change." My husband and daughter joked that I am Chinese because I move furniture so often.

Clocks are such wonderful Chi' enhancers, they create magic in any environment. When I have difficulty sleeping, I try to regulate my pulse/breathing with the rhythm of a regulator clock on our bedroom wall. We have numerous clocks, all set a few minutes apart. I wouldn't want them all to chime at the same time; how could I hear each one. It drives our daughter nuts, she says so many clocks and I never know what time it is here. If you are stressed, then go to a clock shop. I guarantee you will come out feeling better.

First and foremost:

- Honor yourself and facilitate changes to bring people and objects into harmony

- Trust your intuition. Open your Feng Shui eyes

- Increase your vitality. Revitalization is so important for mental, physical and spiritual health, happiness and harmony, peace, tranquility and serenity

- Make personal changes to nurture, protect and support your personal growth

- Be truthful to life's process

- Expect things to flow smoothly all the time

- Expect to be in the right place at the right time

Surviving Caregiving

Addendum 4

Taking Care of Business

We were blessed that we had taken care of all decisions related to one of our end of life decisions. I firmly believe that every family needs to address these issues before they are needed.

It is not 'doom and gloom' – it is a fact of life. I have seen too many people die unexpectedly and distraught family members forced to deal with making decisions, not knowing what loved ones really wanted.

There are many important questions to be answered prior to end of life. Family members need to partake in these discussions/decisions to minimize family dissension.

Taking care of business for end of life issues:

• What are the patient's wishes?

• Is there a trust designating what decisions will be made?

• Who is the designated decision maker?

• Does the patient want CPR, feeding tubes, IV's, invasive procedures, or extensive diagnostic difficult tests/x-ray, CT scans if death is inevitable?

- Or does the patient want comfort only?

- Do you have or want DNRs (Do Not Resuscitate)? Who makes this decision if the patient is unable to? Is it written?

   NOTE: Religious institutions or healthcare providers may be hesitant to comply. Have this conversation early and make certain that everyone understands the patient's wishes.

- Advanced directives need to be current and all healthcare providers need to know the patient's wishes

- Durable power of attorney

- Medical power of attorney or health care proxy

- Is the family able to care for the patient at home? A lot comes into play here

- Does the family have the knowledge and mental, physical, emotional capability to deal with "end of life" stages?

- What are back up options: extended family, friends?

- Does the patient and family want hospice or palliative care? This is an emotional "land mind" for the loved ones. Even if you think you are prepared. Fatigue, anger, frustrations make this a very difficult period

- Will the agency provide 24/7 "in home care" or do

others need to be hired for care? Family respites?

- Is there long term insurance to cover this?

- Is the patient a veteran?

- In 2011, if the patient has a 70% plus disability then palliative care may be available if you live close to a large VA hospital

- The VSO (Veteran's Service Coordinator) or the palliative care supervisor can assist with this transition. Do this early, the process can be cumbersome

- What agency will provide 'durable medical equipment' i.e., hospital beds, oxygen, commodes, etc. How is this paid for?

- Is there a file with vital info? Re: the patient?

- DOB, place of birth, SSN, retirement info – what agencies need to be contacted for benefits? Where is this filed?

- Is there life insurance? Where is it filed? Who is the beneficiary?

Post death:

- Where will the body go, what arrangements need to be made, and is it paid for? Verify all of this ahead of time to make sure it is current

- Do they provide the death certificates (DC's)?

- Do they notify social security? If not be prepared for a 40 minute taped interview. You must have the DC's

- Funeral arrangements

- Death certificates must be received before the legal process starts

- If the body is donated for medical research, that institution will pick up the body and provide the DC's for a fee

- Death certificates: Online at Vital check (www.vitalchek) or 877 459 1069 (current in 2011)

If the decedent is a veteran the VSO will assist with:

- Funeral honors

- Forms completion

- Payment/burial info

If the decedent is a veteran

- Contact DFAS (Defense Finance & Acct Service) to stop benefits. YOU WILL HAVE TO REPAY ALL MONIES RECEIVED AFTER THE DECEDENTS DEATH

All agencies will require:

- Death Certificate

- Date of birth

- Date of death

- Social Security Number

- Some require marriage certificates

  All insurance companies require the death certificates.

- Questions – Where are the policies, what is the process & timeframe for payment?

  Make sure everything is 'Joint custody' if you are married, both spouses must be listed on all accounts.

- Household bills, utilities, credit cards, cell phones

- Property – trusts to prevent family issues, probate

- Loans and who to contact: If the decedent paid, then you will have to make other arrangements

- Bank accts, access numbers. Are they in the trust, who is the beneficiary?

- Cars. Decedent's driver's license for DMV

Surviving Caregiving

Addendum 5

Dealing with the VA Healthcare System

Practical concerns when dealing with the VA Healthcare System.

- As in all medical issues – if it's not documented, it did not happen

- I learned that if I did the research/work for them, i.e. writing out exactly what is needed and presenting it the right way. I would usually get what was needed

- There are never any guarantees. The VA system is flooded with applicants for disabilities these days, so your guess is as good as mine as to the results. I have never been an advocate for "disabilities", broken down it is DIS-ABILITY"

- If you are navigating the healthcare system, find a compassion- ate nurse to assist you with understanding the terminology and the system. You will be the loser if you expect your physician to do this for you

- Physicians practice medicine, but no matter how empathetic, they do not have the skill set to assist you or your family with this process. Do not be bashful. You and your loved ones deserve quality comprehensive health care. That is what you pay for, or in John's case, for what he gave 22 years of his life

• It is important for a caregiver to understand their loved one's diagnosis. Always ask as many questions as needed

• Be persistent and get copies of all of your medical treatment, labs, X-rays and all other procedures. These belong to you. You may have to pay for copies, but historical medical data is so important. DO NOT RELY ON THE MEDICAL SYSTEM TO KEEP THE COPIES OF YOUR RECORDS OR TRANSFER THEM TO OTHER PROVIDERS

Today, more than ever, you have to be proactive. You are in charge of your health. I have seen to many horror stories of not being able to get records for comparison if they are needed later.

Surviving Caregiving

Paperback Available at:
Amazon.com
Your local bookstore

Digital Book Available as:
Amazon Kindle
Barnes and Noble Nook
Apple iBook – Coming soon

http://www.xplica.biz/jotcg

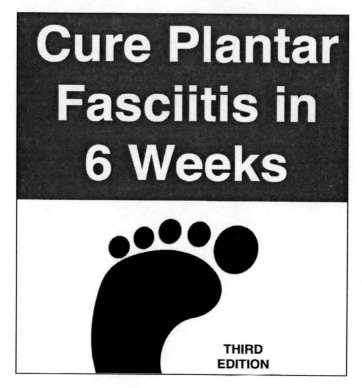

Paperback, Kindle, Nook, iBook
www.xplica.biz/gdfl

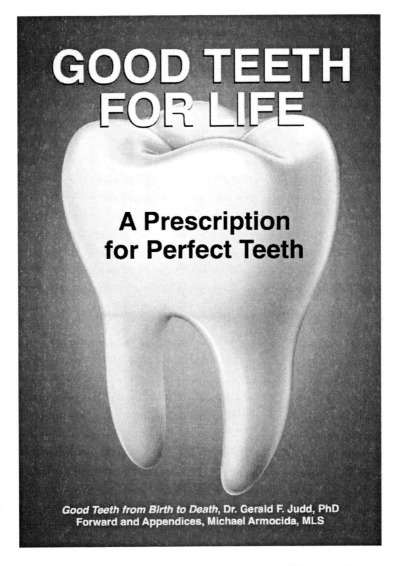

Nearly all animals keep their teeth well into old age.
Why is modern man an exception?

Grammar Quick Reference Sheet
Only $2.99 at Amazon.com

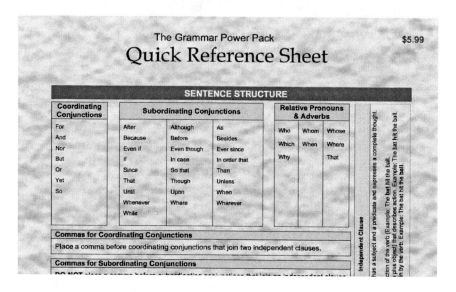

This two-sided laminated sheet is ideal for aspiring writers, students, and business people who want their written work to appear professional and polished. Single glance charts are used as an alternative to remembering the rules of grammar and punctuation. The $2.99 price is discounted from $5.99 to help compensate for Amazon's standard $3.99 shipping costs. Total cost to consumer for item + shipping is estimated at $6.98. American English

www.amazon.com/English-Grammar-Quick-Reference-Sheet/dp/1630419575/?tag=xpl08-20

Coming Soon
www.xplica.biz/pcpp

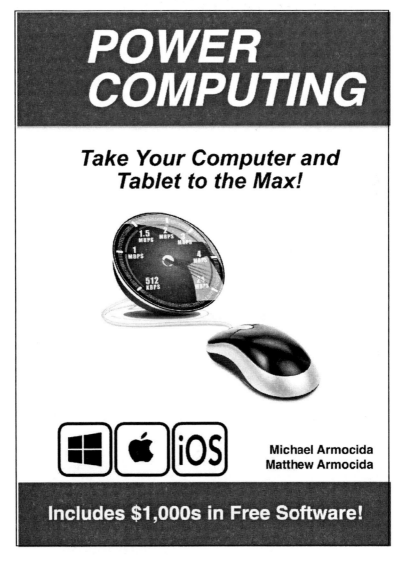
Everything you need to use your computer to the max and do what you never thought possible.